Clinical Methods and Practicum in Speech-Language Pathology

Clinical Methods and Practicum in Speech-Language Pathology

M. N. Hegde
Deborah Davis

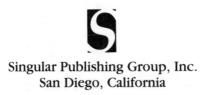

Singular Publishing Group, Inc.
San Diego, California

Singular Textbook Series
Series Editor: M. N. Hegde, Ph.D.

Child Phonology: A Book of Exercises for Students
by Ken Bleile, Ph.D.

Clinical Methods and Practicum in Speech-Language Pathology
by M. N. Hegde, Ph.D., and Deborah Davis, M.A.

Applied Phonetics: The Sounds of American English
by Harold T. Edwards, Ph.D.

Applied Phonetics Workbook: A Systematic Approach to Phonetic Transcription
by Harold T. Edwards, Ph.D., and Alvin L. Gregg, Ph.D.

Teacher's Manual for Applied Phonetics
by Harold T. Edwards, Ph.D.

Also Available

A Singular Manual of Textbook Preparation
by M. N. Hegde

Singular Publishing Group, Inc.
4284 41st Street
San Diego, California 92105

© 1992 by Singular Publishing Group, Inc.

Library of Congress Cataloging-in-Publication Data

Hegde, M. N. (Mahabalagiri N.), 1941–
    Clinical methods and practicum in speech-language pathology / M. N. Hegde, Deborah Davis.
      p.   cm.
    Includes index.
    ISBN 1-879105-42-X
    1. Speech therapy — Study and teaching.   I. Davis, Deborah. 1951–.
  II. Title.
RC428.H44   1991
606.85'506—dc20

            91-26886
            CIP

ISBN 1-879105-42-X

Printed in the United States of America

Contents

Preface

Students who are about to enter clinical practicum in speech-language pathology often are unsure of its organization, scope, and various requirements. Instructors and clinical supervisors consider students who have completed preclinic requirements ready for clinical practicum. Typically, though, these preclinic requirements are academic courses in which little information is offered about the practicum experience itself. Therefore, many students who are about to enroll in clinical practicum do not know how this experience is structured, and what organizational, ethical, and professional rules of service and conduct must be followed.

Students know that practicum involves more than a knowledge of assessment and treatment procedures. They have heard senior friends in the department talk about administrative rules, different practicum sites, writing reports, scheduling clients, meeting with their supervisors, code of ethics, and other matters about which they have little information. Partly because of this lack of knowledge, many students are apprehensive about clinical practice. Therefore, we wrote this text to help students better prepare themselves for the practicum by learning about the organization and functioning of clinical practicum. Though this is intended as a text or reference book for clinical practicum, those who read this ahead of their enrollment in practicum may enter it with less apprehension.

We have organized the book into two parts. Part I gives an overview of clinical practicum, its structure, and function. We have described how the clinical practicum is organized, what activities are involved, what rules and regulations the students must follow, and what they can expect from their supervisors.

Part II gives an overview of the essential treatment methods. We have concentrated on basic treatment methods that apply to all disorders of communication. We expect students to have academic knowledge on which the methods are based. We hope students will find this book a source for quick review of terms and techniques as they prepare for and implement treatment programs for their clients.

We wrote both parts of the text from a practical standpoint. Therefore, including only a few reference citations, we have avoided discussion of research and theories that are handled in academic textbooks. Throughout the book, we have emphasized that clinical practicum is a learning experience and that it is a means of becoming a competent clinician who offers quality service.

We recognize that universities organize their practicum differently and that those differences among programs are often their strengths. Also, individual clinical supervisors shape unique practicum experiences for their students. Therefore, we will be satisfied if clinical supervisors and student clinicians find this book a source of information they can expand and build on. We welcome comments from clinical supervisors who may wish to point out unique procedures or additional matters that may be included in a future edition of this book.

Part I

Clinical Practicum in Speech-Language Pathology

W hen you have completed certain courses in communicative disorders, your advisor may tell you that you are ready for clinical practicum. This means that you have acquired some basic knowledge about communication and its disorders. Yet, you may not know much about the practicum itself. Therefore, in Part I of the text, we have described the organization of clinical practicum, various rules and regulations you must follow, relationship with your clinical supervisor, and some basic principles of working with clients. Read this part of the text carefully to understand what practicum is and how to prepare yourself for it.

In Part II of the text, we have described the basic clinical methods of treating clients with communicative disorders. We have given an overview of commonly used treatment techniques with an emphasis on working with families of your clients to achieve maintenance of treatment gains.

Part I

Clinical Practicum in Speech-Language Pathology

1

Clinical Practicum in Speech-Language Pathology

S peech-language pathology is a profession with scientific and academic bases. To be a speech-language pathologist, you need to gain both academic and scientific knowledge through course work and practical experience in working with clients who have communicative disorders. Therefore, speech-language pathology degree programs at colleges and universities include two types of training.

The first type of training is offered through academic course work. You learn about speech, language, communication, and communicative disorders by taking various academic courses. Some academic courses are a prerequisite to beginning clinical practicum, while others may be taken in conjunction with clinical practicum. The academic portion of the training program gives the student a theoretical basis and foundation for clinical practicum.

The second type of training is offered through clinical practicum. Clinical practicum gives students the opportunity to apply and practice what they have learned in academic courses. The combination of academic course work and practicum provides students with well-rounded training in speech-language pathology.

Occasionally, students try to rate the importance of academic classes versus practicum assignments. However, there is no comparison because each is equally important. Without a strong academic background, students would not know how to assess and treat people with communicative disorders. Without practicum, students would not learn the skills they must have to be successful speech-language pathologists. Therefore, from the beginning, avoid making judgments in favor of one or the other and apply yourself fully and equally to your academic courses and practicum assignments.

Clinical Practicum: An Overview

Clinical practicum is a supervised experience in which students learn professional skills of assessing and treating people with communicative disorders. This experience is designed to prepare students for their future roles as professional speech-language pathologists. Enrollment in clinical practicum is a required part of the curriculum in programs accredited by the American-Speech-Language-Hearing Association (ASHA). Clinical practicum provides the student with the necessary opportunities to apply and expand on the information learned in academic courses.

Students generally enroll in clinical practicum during their senior year as an undergraduate or during their first semester as a graduate student. In some universities, students are allowed to participate in clinical practicum earlier in the training program. This experience may be limited to observing graduate students providing clinical services and assisting with a client or two toward the end of the semester. For example, you may be assigned to observe a student clinician for a semester prior to being assigned your own clients. You will be involved gradually in the treatment process. You may be required to assist in charting responses, developing stimulus materials, and eventually working with the client for one or two sessions as the primary clinician.

As much as the university clinic's caseload allows, the beginning student clinician is assigned clients with less complex disorders. In most universities, student clinicians are assigned clients based on the academic courses they have completed or are enrolled in. For example, during your first semester of graduate work, you may enroll in a course in articulation and be assigned articulation clients only. As you complete course work on other disorders of communication, you may be assigned clients with different types of disorders.

Other universities take a more gestalt viewpoint of clinical experience and provide the student clinician with a variety of clients each term, based on the student's individual level of expertise, previous educational experience, and the supervisor's expertise. For example, as a first semester graduate student, you may take a seminar in articulation, a seminar in language, and a seminar in research methods. However, in your clinical practicum, you may be assigned a fluency client based on your undergraduate class in fluency and the expertise of your clinical supervisor.

You will participate in clinical practicum assignments at both the university clinic and various off-campus clinical sites. Many universities require that student clinicians complete a certain minimum number of clinical hours before they are assigned to off-campus practicum sites. Your clinical practicum may include hospital, school, or various other clinical sites.

You are given more responsibility in planning, evaluating, and treating clients as you progress through your clinical and academic programs. As a beginning student clinician, you will not be expected to have all the answers; your clinical supervisor will help you find those answers. As you gain clinical experience, you will be expected to perform more independently in most of your clinical responsibilities.

General Preclinic Requirements

In addition to a solid academic foundation, good writing skills are necessary for success in clinical practicum. Equally important is your ability to talk to people from all walks of life and of all ages. Finally, there are less tangible, personal characteristics without which you cannot successfully complete your clinical practicum. You are not expected to enter clinical practicum with all the necessary skills, but you should be able to learn from your experiences and interactions with your supervisor.

Academic Requirements

Preclinic academic requirements are completed both at the under-graduate and graduate levels. At the undergraduate level, you probably will take courses on phonetics, anatomy and physiology of speech and hearing mechanisms, speech science (perception and production of speech), and those related to normal acquisition of speech and language. Some clinical courses, especially those related to disorders of articulation, language, voice, fluency, and hearing also may be taken at the undergraduate level.

Graduate courses give you more advanced information on all aspects of communicative disorders, their assessment, and treatment. These courses are more research based than the undergraduate courses. Graduate courses build on the information offered at the undergraduate level and emphasize specialized information. For example, besides taking advanced courses in articulation and language, you also take courses in stuttering, aphasia, cleft palate, augmentative communication, and neurologically based speech disorders.

Although course requirements and sequences vary from university to university, students are expected to have minimally completed introductory courses in normal and abnormal speech and language development and introductory courses in speech and hearing science before beginning clinical practicum. You should discuss the specific requirements with your advisor well in advance of the time you plan to begin your clinical practicum.

General Writing Requirements

Student clinicians are required to write numerous clinical reports, treatment programs, lesson plans, and progress notes. Therefore, it is important that you develop your writing skills prior to your enrollment in clinical practicum. You are not expected to know the specific formats for reports and some of the technical terms prior to clinical enrollment, but you should be able to write clearly and concisely. You should be able to organize your thoughts coherently and write grammatically correct sentences. Your writing should be free from spelling errors.

If you are concerned about your general writing skills, discuss your problem with your advisor as early in your program as possible. Your advisor can assist you in overcoming your writing problems. You may need to take a writing course, or you may need just additional practice in writing. These and other steps will prepare you for meeting clinical writing requirements.

Personal Characteristics

In addition to academic preparation and good writing skills, students preparing to enroll in clinical practicum should be aware of the personal characteristics required for successful clinical work. Probably one of the most important characteristics is responsible behavior.

Student clinicians are expected to act responsibly in all areas of clinical involvement including preparation for treatment sessions, meeting with clients, report writing, and interactions with office staff and clinical supervisors. You will have deadlines for various clinical assignments including scheduling of clients, completion of various reporting forms needed by the clinic administrative staff, and submission of diagnostic reports, treatment plans, and lesson plans. It is understood that you must be prepared in advance for each diagnostic and treatment session for which you are scheduled.

Student clinicians also need to develop the ability to work independently within their level of experience. For example, as a beginning clinician you are expected to rely on your supervisor for assistance more than experienced clinicians do; however, you still must be prepared to research material independently and, with your supervisor's help, evaluate the efficacy of your clinical sessions, determine areas of needed change, and implement appropriate modifications that your supervisor suggests to you. Student clinician's responsibilities are discussed in more detail in chapter 4.

Knowledge of the Profession and Related Agencies

Students preparing to enroll in clinical practicum should have at least a basic knowledge of the various accrediting and licensing agencies and regulations related to the profession of speech-language pathology. Two agencies affect your training and professional career the most: The American-Speech-Language-Hearing Association (ASHA); and, if your state has a licensure law, the Board of Examiners for Audiology and Speech Pathology (or other licensing agency in your state) .

The American-Speech-Language-Hearing Association. Students and student clinicians in departments of communicative disorders or speech-language pathology will repeatedly hear references to ASHA and ASHA's requirements. Student clinicians will constantly be told of ASHA's requirements on how to complete their clinical practicum.

As you probably know, ASHA is a scientific and professional organization with a long history of contributions to communicative disorders. This national organization is the major force that shapes our scientific and professional discipline. The organization acts as an advocate for individuals with communicative disorders and the professionals who provide services to these individuals. ASHA has five primary goals.

1. The maintenance of high standards of clinical competence for speech-language pathology and audiology services provided to the public.
2. The development of comprehensive clinical service programs.
3. The investigation of clinical procedures used in treatment of communicative disorders.
4. The research and study of human communication and its disorders.
5. The exchange of ideas and information about communicative disorders through various continuing professional education activities (ASHA Membership and Certification Handbook, 1990).

ASHA works in various ways to maintain high standards of clinical competence. It sponsors conferences and workshops to encourage continuing professional education. ASHA collects and disseminates data related to research, clinical service delivery, education, and career opportunities. It has established accreditation and certification procedures that outline minimal standards of education and clinical service delivery. These standards are outlined in the form of academic and clinical preparation and include compliance with the ASHA Code of Ethics.

University training programs that meet ASHA standards may receive **accreditation** from ASHA. Individuals completing a program of study and clinical experience approved by ASHA may receive **certification.** This certification is known as the **Certificate of Clinical Competence**, and more commonly referred to as the **CCC.** This certificate may be in audiology or speech-language pathology. Remember, accreditation is awarded to programs, while certification is awarded to individuals.

ASHA accredits academic programs and clinical services through two of its agencies. **Educational Standards Board (ESB)** accredits academic programs and **Professional Services Board (PSB)** accredits the clinical services. A university must request accreditation of its academic program, its clinical services, or both. The university may seek accreditation for its speech-language pathology program, audiology program, or both. ASHA will then send a team of experts to evaluate the educational programs and another team to evaluate the clinical services offered by the university. ASHA accredits only master's degree programs.

The team evaluating educational programs looks at the quality and number of faculty teaching the courses, the curriculum offered by the department, the library and other resources of the university, and many other factors that affect the education of future speech-language pathologists and audiologists.

The team evaluating clinical services offered by the department looks at the qualifications and certification status of clinical supervisors, adequacy of physical facilities and clinical equipment, and all other factors that affect the quality of clinical services offered to the public. Each team submits a report to the ASHA Board they are responsible for (ESB or PSB). Based on these reports, the ESB and the PSB will make a final decision on whether to accredit the program.

Both ESB and PSB requirements directly influence you and your training program. First, if you are attending a program accredited by ASHA, you are assured that the department has met ASHA's standards. Second, beginning January 1, 1994, an individual must have graduated from an ESB accredited program to be eligible for the Certificate of Clinical Competence.

As you now know, the Certificate of Clinical Competence (CCC) is awarded by ASHA to individuals who have successfully met ASHA's academic, clinical, and ethical standards in speech-language pathology, audiology, or both. To be eligible for certification, an individual must satisfy several requirements.

First, individuals applying for certification prior to January 1, 1993 must hold a master's degree or equivalent in speech-language pathology or audiology. The equivalency requirement is met when a person does not have a master's degree, but has completed at least 30 units of graduate work in speech-language pathology or audiology. Individuals applying for certification January 1, 1993 or later must hold a master's or doctoral degree in speech-language pathology. Equivalent course work without a master's degree will no longer satisfy the minimum requirement for certification (ASHA Council on Professional Standards in Speech-Language Pathology & Audiology, 1991).

Second, after completing the educational and clinical requirements at the college level, individuals are required to complete a **Clinical Fellowship Year (CFY)**. The CFY consists of paid (or volunteer) experience supervised by a professional holding current ASHA certification in the same area in which certification is sought (speech-language pathology or audiology). The CFY can be completed in 9 months of full-time work (at least 30 hours per week) or up to 36 months of part-time work (15–19 hours per week). Note that less than 15 hours of work per week does not meet ASHA's CFY requirements. The CFY requirement is not part of the university's clinical training program. Its purpose is to help the individual bridge the gap between student practicum and independent professional practice (ASHA Membership & Certification Handbook, 1990).

Third, candidates for the CCC must obtain a passing score on the **National Examination in Speech-Language Pathology and Audiology (NESPA)**. The NESPA is a comprehensive assessment of an individual's knowledge in the area of speech-language pathology or audiology. The examination consists of objective questions. The NESPA can usually be taken through your university's testing office.

Fourth, all individuals (students and graduates) seeking ASHA certification must agree to abide by the ASHA Code of Ethics. Chapter 3 contains a more detailed discussion of the code of ethics.

Fifth, a membership fee must be submitted with the application for certification. ASHA publishes a **Membership and Certification Handbook** which contains application forms as well as detailed information regarding academic, practicum, CFY, and membership requirements. Contact ASHA to obtain this handbook.

Although the CCC does not confirm any legal status, it is recognized as a necessary requisite for practice in most employment settings excluding public schools. Many state licensure requirements are based on the CCC requirements.

Licensure Board. Depending on where you live and what setting you practice in, you also may need to meet state licensure and credentialing requirements. In states that have a licensure law, ASHA's CCC is not sufficient to practice speech-language pathology or audiology.

Licensure is regulated by a state government agency (e.g., Board of Examiners for Audiology and Speech Pathology). The majority of states in the United States now have licensure requirements for speech-language pathologists. With the exception of only a few states, the state licensure requirements are compatible with those of CCC. Many states also have licensure reciprocity with the CCC (Lynch, 1990). Commonly exempt from licensure requirements are speech-language pathologists providing services in the public schools or federal government agencies.

Department of Education. The speech-language pathologist who plans to work in the public schools must obtain an educational credential or certificate issued by the state's department of education.

To practice speech-language services in the schools, the clinician need not have the state licensure or ASHA's CCC; but many would like to have them anyway. Educational and practicum requirements of most educational credentials are similar to those of CCC and state licensure. However, there may be some unique requirements for the educational credential that vary across states.

In addition to the course work required for your master's degree, a student seeking a school credential often needs to take courses related to public school speech, language, and hearing programs. Additional courses related to public school education also may be required. A student internship in the school setting is a typical credentialing requirement.

Several states offer more than one educational credential for speech-language pathologists. With some credentials, you may be able to teach students who are or who are not communicatively handicapped. With other credentials, you may be able to offer clinical services and teach all subjects to a special group of children who are handicapped. Clinicians who do not wish to be teachers seek a credential that allows them to work individually or in small groups with children with communicative disorders. Each state has its own educational credential laws for the speech-language pathologist. Because of this diversity and unique educational requirements for public school credentials in different states, you must consult with your advisor early in your clinical training. As you continue in your training program, you will become more familiar with the various requirements in your state.

The National Student Speech-Language-Hearing Association.

An excellent source of professional information in your department might be the local chapter of the **National Student Speech-Language-Hearing Association (NSSLHA)**. Local chapters of NSSLHA are run by students with the help of a faculty advisor. The NSSLHA is a national organization affiliated with ASHA, and its main purpose is to help students enrolled in speech-language pathology and audiology programs get involved with their future profession.

Your local chapter is an association of supportive fellow students who organize fund-raising activities, social events, and professional workshops and seminars. Therefore, early in your undergraduate program, become a member of the local chapter of NSSLHA. This membership will help you keep current with all aspects of your profession.

NSSLHA membership dues are a fraction of the ASHA dues, and yet you receive many of the same benefits offered to full dues-paying professional members of ASHA. Members of NSSLHA receive all ASHA journals. These journals are a valuable source of scientific and professional information you cannot do without. As a graduate student, you will appreciate having your own collection of journals which you frequently will be asked to read. NSSLHA also publishes its own journal, which is distributed to its members. NSSLHA members are eligible to attend certain state and national conferences at reduced rates. Besides, NSSLHA gives students the opportunity to begin developing a social and professional network with individuals with similar interests.

ASHA Guidelines on Practicum

To ensure that students receive a broad but comprehensive training program, ASHA has established guidelines on clinical practicum. You satisfy the clinical practicum and internship requirements by showing that you have enough clinical clock hours earned under the supervision of an ASHA certified speech-language pathologist or audiologist. ASHA mandates requirements for both students and supervisors. This section of the text emphasizes the requirements for students.

Clinical Observation

Clinical observation offers students a nonthreatening introduction to the clinical process. It allows you to begin your preparation for clinical practicum by observing the work of more experienced clinicians. Observation is your opportunity to find out how what you have learned through your academic course work is applied in the clinic. By observing other clinicians, you begin to understand the assessment and treatment process.

ASHA requires students to obtain a minimum of 25 clock hours of supervised clinical observation before they begin their clinical practicum. Most students will observe live clinical sessions. However, observation of videotaped sessions or of live sessions on closed-circuit television monitors is also acceptable.

Observation hours may be obtained for treatment and evaluation of individuals with communicative disorders. Observations may be of children or adults. The 25 hours may be a combination of audiology and speech-language pathology observation; it is not 25 hours of audiology or 25 hours of speech-language pathology. However, many universities specify that students' majority of observation hours be obtained in their area of professional emphasis (speech-language pathology or audiology). Other universities require a fairly equal distribution of observation hours between speech-language pathology and audiology. Regardless of the required distribution of observation hours, the 25 hours are a minimum requirement, and additional observation hours are strongly advised.

You must observe services provided by individuals who currently are certified by ASHA in speech-language pathology or audiology. You also may observe other student clinicians who are supervised by individuals holding current ASHA certification. Observation hours are verified by reviewing your observation log and observation reports.

While it is appropriate to observe the same client over a period of time to note the progression of treatment, you also should sample a variety of clients and disorders. You should observe both children and adults being evaluated and treated.

To maximize the observation experience, you should be prepared to take notes and describe specific components of a session. If possible, review the client's file or discuss the session with the clinician prior to observing. Ideally, after you have completed an observation, you should be able to answer the following questions.

1. What type of communicative disorder did the client exhibit?
2. What were the objectives of the session?
3. What were the target behaviors?
4. How was the session structured? (e.g., Was there an introduction and a closing segment to the session?)
5. How was the room arranged?
6. How were the client and the clinician seated in relation to each other?
7. What types of materials and activities were used?
8. What did the clinician do to teach the target behaviors?
9. How were undesirable behaviors decreased?
10. How were responses charted?

Responsibilities of Student Observers. Remember, student observers are representatives of the university and are expected to demonstrate responsible and ethical behavior. When observing at both on- and off-campus sites, you should comply with the following guidelines.

1. **Arrive on time for observations.** If you arrive late for a scheduled observation you may disrupt the evaluation or treatment session. You also will not have a chance to discuss the client with the clinician prior to the session. If you do not know how the sessions started, you may have trouble understanding what you observe. Arriving late for a scheduled observation is irresponsible behavior. Clinical supervisors may not allow late arrivals to observe the session.

2. **When you arrive at your observation session, introduce yourself to the clinical supervisor and request permission to observe.** Although the observation may have been scheduled previously, there now may be reasons that prohibit the observation. For example, the client may have, for whatever reason, decided against being observed; the clinical supervisor may have determined that the observation area was too crowded, or that the observation would not be beneficial for you or the client.

3. **To obtain the greatest benefit from your observation, observe the entire clinical session.** Each treatment and evaluation session has a continuum that must be followed. If you arrive late or leave early, you will not be able to see this progression.

4. **Always respect the client's right to confidentiality.** Never discuss your observations with individuals outside the clinic setting. If you have a report to make regarding your observation, you may refer to the person observed as "the client" or "the individual."

5. **Do not discuss a client by name except in conversation with the client's clinician or clinical supervisor.** In this case, discuss the client only when confidentiality is assured. Do not discuss the client when other people who may overhear your conversation are around.

6. **When you talk with the clinician, do not interrupt the session or waste the preparation time he or she has allotted between clients.** This is one more reason why it is important to arrive on time for your observations and to observe entire sessions.

7. **Do not remove clinical files from the clinic area.** In most cases, you will be able to review the client's file to obtain background information. While reviewing the files, do not write in them, remove anything from the files, or take notes.

8. **Increase your observation skills by phonetically transcribing utterances, charting correct and incorrect productions, and noting test results.** The time you spend

observing is for your benefit. The more you learn during your observations, the more skills and confidence you will have to bring to your first practicum experience.

9. **After your observation, complete an observation report form for each client.** Request the clinical supervisor to sign the observation report. Without a signature, observation hours may not be valid. Observation reports should be turned into the clinic director or clinical supervisor. These reports will be used to substantiate your observation hours prior to your admittance to clinical practicum.

10. **Present yourself as a professional.** There will be clients, family members of the client, and other professionals at your observation site. You need to dress and behave like a professional. Therefore, be sure to follow the clinic dress code. Professional attire is considered appropriate dress. If you have doubts as to whether something is appropriate to wear, do not wear it.

Various clinical sites may have additional rules and procedures. It is your responsibility to know the guidelines for observers at your site. It is also your responsibility to follow ASHA's Code of Ethics during clinical observations. The Code of Ethics is described in chapter 3.

Clinical Practicum

After you have taken the preclinic academic courses and completed supervised clinical observation requirements, you will be able to begin your clinical practicum supervised by an individual who holds a current CCC in speech-language pathology or audiology. Many states have licensure and credential requirements that clinical supervisors must also meet.

Clinical practicum clock hours are earned for screening, evaluation, and treatment of communicative disorders. Regardless of how experienced the student clinician is, a minimum of 25% of treatment sessions and a minimum of 50% of each diagnostic session must be supervised (ASHA Council on Professional Standards in Speech-Language Pathology and Audiology, 1990).

Number of Clinical Clock Hours Required. ASHA's guidelines for completion of the CCC in Speech-Language Pathology *for applications received prior to January 1, 1993* requires the student clinician to earn a minimum of 300 total clock hours with children and adults. These 300 hours must be earned through a combination of the following.

1. A minimum of 200 clock hours earned in speech-language pathology.
2. A minimum of 150 clock hours earned at the graduate level.
3. A minimum of 50 clock hours earned in at least two separate clinical settings.
4. A minimum of 50 clock hours earned in the evaluation of speech and language problems.
5. A minimum of 75 clock hours earned in the treatment of language disorders.
6. A minimum of 25 clock hours earned in the treatment of fluency disorders.
7. A minimum of 25 clock hours earned in the treatment of voice disorders.
8. A minimum of 25 clock hours earned in the treatment of articulation disorders.
9. A minimum of 35 clock hours in audiology. Of these, 15 clock hours must be earned in the area of evaluation and/or treatment of speech-language problems associated with hearing impairments and 15 clock hours in evaluation of auditory disorders. The remaining 5 hours may be earned in either the area of evaluation of auditory disorders or in the area of evaluation or treatment of speech-language problems associated with hearing impairments.
10. Some experience must be earned working with groups.

Guidelines for completion of the CCC in Audiology for *applications received prior to January 1, 1993,* also require earning a minimum of 300 total clock hours with children and adults. These hours must be earned through a combination of the following.

1. A minimum of 200 clock hours completed in audiology.
2. A minimum of 150 clock hours earned at the graduate level.
3. A minimum of 50 clock hours earned in at least two separate clinical settings.
4. A minimum of 50 clock hours in the identification and evaluation of hearing impairment.
5. A minimum of 50 clock hours in the habilitation or rehabilitation of individuals with hearing impairments.
6. A minimum of 35 clock hours in speech-language pathology. These hours are evaluation and treatment of speech and language problems not related to hearing impairment.

Individuals submitting applications for the Certificate of Clinical Competence in Speech-Language Pathology postmarked January 1, 1993 or after must comply with the new academic and clinical standards adopted by ASHA October 23, 1988. These standards require students to complete a minimum of 375 clock hours that include the following.

1. A minimum of 25 supervised clinical observation hours.
2. A minimum of 350 total clinical practicum clock hours with a total of 250 of the hours earned at the graduate level in the area in which the certificate is sought (audiology or speech-language pathology).
3. A minimum of 50 clock hours earned in each of three types of clinical settings. The clinical settings must offer distinctly different clinical experiences, but may or may not be within the same institution. For example, the university may have special voice and augmentative communication clinics. Though they are located at the same address, they offer unique clinical experiences. Public schools and hospitals also may provide more than a single clinical experience. You also may participate in practicum at three or more different locations. For instance, your practicum may include assignment at an acute care hospital, a public school, and your university clinic.
4. A minimum of 20 evaluation hours in each of the following categories: speech disorders in children, speech disorders in adults, language disorders in children, and language disorders in adults.
5. A minimum of 20 treatment hours in each of the following: speech disorders in children, speech disorders in adults, language disorders in children, language disorders in adults.
6. A minimum of 35 hours in audiology. Of these 35 hours, 15 hours are required in the evaluation or screening of auditory disorders, and 15 hours are required in the habilitation or rehabilitation of individuals with auditory disorders. The remaining 5 hours may be earned in either evaluation of auditory disorders or in the area of habilitation or rehabilitation of individuals with auditory disorders (ASHA Council on Professional Standards in Speech-Language Pathology & Audiology, 1991).

Students also may earn up to 20 clock hours in a related disorder. These hours may include a variety of experiences. For example, activities may be related to the improvement of oral pharyngeal function and related disorders, the development and conservation of optimal communication, or the prevention of speech or language disorders. These hours are optional.

Individuals applying for the CCC in Audiology on or after January 1, 1993 must meet ASHA's new guidelines on academic and clinical standards. A total of 375 clinical clock hours are required. Briefly, these requirements include the following.

1. A minimum of 25 supervised clinical observation hours.
2. A minimum of 350 clock hours with at least 250 of the hours earned in audiology practicum at the graduate level.
3. A minimum of 50 clock hours earned in each of three types of clinical settings.
4. A minimum of 40 clock hours earned in each of the following categories: evaluation of hearing in children and evaluation of hearing in adults.
5. A minimum of 80 hours must be earned in the selection and use of amplification and assistive devices, with a minimum of 10 hours each with children and adults.
6. A minimum of 20 clock hours earned in the treatment of hearing disorders in children and adults.
7. A minimum of 35 clock hours in speech-language pathology. These hours must be unrelated to hearing impairment and include 15 hours in evaluation or screening and 15 hours in treatment. The remaining 5 hours may be in evaluation, screening, or treatment (ASHA Council on Professional Standards, 1991).

As part of the 350 practicum hours, audiology students may earn up to 20 clock hours in related disorders. For instance, students may earn hours for activities related to hearing conservation programs (ASHA Council on Professional Standards in Speech-Language Pathology & Audiology, 1991).

The total clock hours required by ASHA are the minimum number of practicum hours. Your department may have additional practicum hour requirements. Check with your advisor to ensure that you meet the requirements of ASHA and your university.

What to Count As Clinical Clock Hours.   Sometimes there is confusion on what types of activities can be counted as clinical clock hours and what category the clock hours should be counted under. Use the following guidelines in recording your clock hours.

1. **Clock hours may be earned in conjunction with a class assignment and during clinical practicum.** For example,

if as part of a class assignment in a course on aphasia, you are required to evaluate a client with aphasia, you may earn diagnostic clock hours even when not enrolled in clinical practicum. However, to earn those hours, you must be supervised by an individual who holds a CCC in speech-language pathology. Also, a minimum of 50% of the evaluation must have been supervised by that individual.

2. **Diagnostic hours are earned for both screening and assessments of communicative disorders.** Typically, the student clinician may earn screening hours at local preschools, at area public and private schools, at health fairs, and at the university clinic. Speech, language, and hearing screenings also may be performed at facilities serving the elderly. Diagnostic hours may be earned while you are enrolled in a section of the clinic designated solely for evaluations. You may also acquire diagnostic hours as part of the assessment of your clients at the beginning of the treatment period. Readministering specific tests or other assessment procedures at the end of treatment to document the status of the client also may be counted as evaluation hours. However, administering probes during the treatment period should not be counted as diagnostic hours. Time spent administering probes can be counted with treatment hours.

3. **Clock hours are earned for counseling clients or counseling or training family members.** Such counseling, of course, is closely relative to the communicative disorder of a client. For example, providing treatment for a client with a diagnosis of aphasia might include not only direct language intervention with the client, but sharing information with the client's family. It might be necessary for you to explain to the family members what aphasia means and how they can help the client regain some of the lost communicative behaviors. Or, your articulation treatment for a preschool child might include a home training program. In that case, you need to train the parents to ensure that they are able to carry out the home assignments

4. **Clock hours are credited for the time spent in obtaining or giving assessment and treatment information.** You can count the time you spend taking a case history, interviewing the client, the client's family, or both. You can also count the time you spend discussing your diagnosis and recommendations with the client or client's family.

5. **Clock hours are earned for treatment and evaluation of a variety of disorders.** For example, clock hours earned in

language treatment may include treatment of individuals with aphasia, language delay, or traumatic brain injury. Hours earned in articulation may include treatment provided for individuals with apraxia, dysarthria, phonological disorders, or dialect modification. Hours earned in voice disorders may include treatment of individuals with dysarthria or treatment of pitch, intensity, or resonance disorders. Time spent treating individuals with laryngectomy or hearing impairments also may be counted under voice. Hours earned in fluency may include time spent treating individuals with any type of disordered rhythm. Individuals applying for certification January 1, 1993 or later count hours earned in articulation, voice, and fluency disorders under the category of speech disorders.

6. **If a client has more than one type of communicative disorder, you can count separately the time spent in treating each disorder.** A child with a cleft palate may have disordered articulation, voice, and language. An individual with dysarthria may present both an articulation and a voice disorder. An individual with aphasia may have concomitant apraxia. An individual with a hearing impairment may have an articulation, voice, and language disorder. In all such cases, divide your clock hours according to how much time was spent in diagnosing or treating each of the disorders.

7. **Clinical staffings may be counted as clock hours if you are applying for ASHA certification after January 1, 1993.** Clinical staffings may include activities such as meetings with other professionals to discuss your client's treatment. However, your meetings with your clinical supervisor to discuss treatment plans and procedures cannot be counted as clinical staffings. A maximum of 25 clock hours may be acquired from participation in client staffings with or without the client present when evaluation, treatment, or recommendations are discussed.

8. **Do not count preparation time as clinical clock hours.** Although you will spend much time in gathering materials or ideas, writing reports and lesson plans, scoring tests or transcribing language samples, you cannot count clock hours for these activities.

9. **Do not count inservice or workshop presentations as clock hours.** Your practicum assignment may require you to provide inservice training. For example, in the public school

setting you may be required to make a presentation to the teaching staff regarding the services provided by speech-language pathologists. Although this activitiy is part of a student clinician's responsibility, it may not be counted as clock hours.

Remember that most clinical practicum clock hours are earned for direct client contact time only. The exceptions are the 25 staffing hours that can be counted and counseling and training a client's family directly related to a client's communicative disorder.

Payment for Clinical Services. According to ASHA guidelines, students in clinical practicum are not allowed to receive payment for their services. You may, however, be eligible for other types of financial assistance. Your university may have scholarships, grants, or stipends for which you can apply. Some practicum assignments also provide stipends which are not considered payment for clinical services. Your advisor and the financial aid office at your university can give you information on financial assistance available to you.

Clinical Practicum as a Learning Experience

Clinical practicum is designed to give you an exceptional learning experience. The practicum gives you an opportunity to gain experience with a wide variety of individuals with communicative disorders. Under the supervision of qualified speech-language pathologists, you learn to evaluate and treat clients with fluency, voice, language, and articulation disorders of various severities and etiologies. You will gain experience in many different clinical settings including acute care hospitals, rehabilitation facilities, psychiatric hospitals, skilled nursing facilities, private practices, and public schools.

Initially, you may be somewhat apprehensive about beginning your practicum. This is a normal response, but as you gain more experience and confidence, you will discover that clinical practicum is exciting and rewarding. You are encouraged to experience as many types of clients and clinical settings as you can.

Remember, you are a student and are not expected to perform like an experienced professional. What is expected of you is that you demonstrate consistent progress in each of your practicum assign-ments. Speech-language pathology is exciting partly because there is always something new to learn.

Now you have a general idea of the personal and academic requirements for a successful clinical practicum. You also know ASHA's requirements for types of practicum hours and clinical settings in which to acquire them. This is your chance to apply information learned in academic classes and explore some of the possibilities the profession of speech-language pathology has to offer.

2

Organization of Clinical Practicum

C linical practicum is organized on a hierarchy of clinical experiences and expectations. Clinical practicum begins at the university clinic. Beginning student clinicians are assigned one or two clients. As student clinicians gain experience, become more confident, and are able to make more independent decisions, their client caseload is increased. The clinicians then may be assigned to off campus clinical settings for clinical internships.

The Typical University Clinic

The typical university clinic strives to provide high quality clinical services in conjunction with appropriate educational experiences for student clinicians. The clinic is designed and equipped to facilitate clinical training and promote clinical research.

The university clinical facilities are arranged to maximize observation of sessions with minimal distractions. Many clinics are equipped with observation windows for viewing and an audio system for listening. Student clinicians providing clinical services at a university clinic should be prepared for frequent observations by supervisors, family members of clients, and other students. Your supervisor may enter the treatment room to observe your session or to demonstrate a specific treatment technique. Your sessions may be videotaped for later observation or class demonstration. Your sessions also may be recorded by a television camera for a closed-circuit television monitor.

Supervision at the university clinic may be provided by the university teaching faculty, full-time supervisory faculty, part-time supervisory staff, or a combination of the three. You may have one supervisor per term or more than one supervisor based on the departmental policy and clinical schedule. Most departments tend to assign a single supervisor to beginning clinicians. All supervision at ASHA accredited universities should be in compliance with the ASHA guidelines on supervision. Accordingly, a minimum of 25% of all treatment sessions are supervised and a minimum of 50% of all diagnostic sessions are supervised by an individual currently certificated in the area in which he or she supervises (speech-language pathology or audiology). The amount of supervision provided also may be adjusted upward depending on your level of clinical experience, the complexity of your client's disorder, or both.

Typically, the university clinic is operated on an 8:00 a.m. to 5:00 p.m. weekday schedule. Some universities also have evening hours to accommodate individuals who cannot attend the clinic during regular business hours. Many university clinics provide services only during the academic year. This schedule disrupts services offered to clients who often need sustained and continuous treatment. To provide more continuous services, some clinics operate 12 months of the year with the professional staff providing services during the intersessions.

Clients usually are scheduled for two to three sessions per week with each session lasting 30 to 60 minutes. Evaluation sessions are sometimes scheduled for larger blocks of time. Most clients are scheduled for individual treatment sessions; however, some clients may be scheduled for group sessions. Generally you will be allotted 5 to 10 minutes between clients to organize your materials. It is important to be sufficiently prepared for your sessions in advance; the few minutes between clients is obviously not the time for planning assessment or treatment activities. This is the time for you to finish with one client and get the next client from the clinic waiting room.

A wide range of ages and communicative disorders are represented in the university clinic's caseload. The university caseload is influenced by demographics and the availability of other speech-language pathology services in the community. For example, if there is a large rehabilitation agency in the area, the clinic may enroll fewer clients with diagnoses of aphasia; if there is a pediatric hospital offering speech and hearing services, the clinic may serve a limited number of children.

Another factor influencing the university client caseload is the expertise of specific faculty members. For instance, if your department has faculty members well known for their expertise in voice disorders, the clinic may attract a large number of clients with voice disorders.

At the beginning of the semester, you will receive your clinical assignment. You will be given your clinic schedule, and your supervisor or clinic director will assign you appropriate clients. At most universities, the student clinician is responsible for telephoning the client and confirming the client's clinic schedule.

Prior to meeting your client, you must review the client's clinical file, develop a plan for the first meeting with your client, and discuss the plan with your clinical supervisor. You should also discuss any evaluation plans with your supervisor and notify your supervisor of the time the evaluation is scheduled.

Your supervisor frequently evaluates your clinical skills. You may get both written and verbal feedback. You may have weekly meetings with your clinical supervisor, weekly staffings, or discussions after each clinical session. At the minimum, you will receive a written final evaluation; most departments provide written midterm evaluations as well. If your progress in the clinical practicum is unsatisfactory, you will be notified and counseled regarding your continued participation in the program.

University clinics have varying policies and terminology regarding writing assignments. Some universities require daily lesson plans, others require weekly lesson plans, and still others require semester treatment plans. You may be required to submit typed plans, handwritten plans, or plans printed on computer printers. Whatever the format, your supervisor will review all your plans. At the end of the term, you will be required to write a progress report or a final summary. The final report should describe the client's status at the beginning of treatment, the treatment goals, the treatment procedures, and the progress made by the client. Your clinical supervisor will give you instructions regarding the format and timelines for all written work.

Off-Campus Practicum Sites

Off-campus practicum sites vary from region to region and from university to university. Common off-campus practicum sites include public schools, hospitals, skilled nursing facilities, rehabilitation agencies, psychiatric hospitals, preschool programs, and private speech and hearing centers.

The first semester (or quarter) of clinical practicum typically is completed in a university speech and hearing clinic. Student clinicians may begin off-campus practicum any time after their first term of clinical practicum. Off-campus practicum usually is supervised by an ASHA-certified speech-language pathologist who works at that site with consultation provided by the university supervisor. All off-campus sites must comply with ASHA's regulations on the frequency and type of supervision.

Student clinicians usually are required to follow the holiday schedule of the off-campus site instead of the schedule of the university. Student clinicians also must comply with the site's requirements regarding professional responsibility and conduct. University grading policy and the department's criteria of acceptable performance dictate the grading.

Public Schools

In many states, to obtain a credential or certificate to provide speech-language pathology services in the public schools, student clinicians must complete a practicum experience in a school setting. The student clinician completes an internship, popularly known as a "student teaching" assignment under the supervision of an appropriately credentialed and ASHA-certified speech-language pathologist employed by the school district. A supervisor from the university training program will coordinate this arrangement.

Student teaching practica generally are full-day assignments, 3 to 5 days a week, perhaps in conjunction with a weekly seminar. The school day usually is from 8:00 a.m. to 4:00 p.m., but you should be prepared to spend additional outside time for writing reports, planning sessions, and preparing materials.

While the practicum provides experience in assessing and treating children who are communicatively handicapped in the school, the seminar held at the university provides a forum for discussing issues and exchanging information. In this seminar, historical and current issues affecting the school speech-language pathologist and the organization and administration of speech-language pathology programs in the public schools may be discussed. Also, student clinicians will have the opportunity to share their practicum experiences and exchange ideas.

Speech-language pathology services in the public schools are designed to meet the needs of all individuals who are communicatively handicapped and eligible for school services as mandated by federal legislation, **The Education for All Handicapped Childrens' Act (EHA), Public Law 94-142 (P.L. 94-142)**. P.L. 94-142 was passed on November 25, 1975 and provided for educational services for all handicapped children (Dublinske & Healey, 1978). Although several amendments to the EHA have been made over the years, it remains the cornerstone for special education services. The discretionary programs of the EHA were reauthorized in 1990. At that time, the name was changed to the Individuals with Disabilities Education Act (IDEA) (ASHA Governmental Affairs Review, 1990).

The EHA Amendments of 1986, P.L. 99-457 (Part H of EHA), established funds for states to provide services for children from birth through 2 years of age who have disabilities. Services to the families of these children were also included in P.L. 99-457. In addition, the 1986 EHA Amendments included legislation (Part B of EHA) on personnel standards. Part B of P.L. 99-457 requires state education agencies to develop and maintain personnel standards based on the highest requirements in the state. For speech-language pathologists, including school speech-language pathologists, this standard is the master's degree (ASHA Congressional Relations Division, Government Affairs Department, 1989).

The school speech-language pathology services are governed by several other federal laws and guidelines. State laws and regulations on special education also affect speech-language pathology services provided in the public schools. School speech-language pathologists must know and follow all guidelines affecting their school sites.

As one might expect from the wide range of ages offered services in the public schools, the caseload for student clinicians participating in clinical practicum in that setting can be varied enough to satisfy almost anyone's professional interests. In addition to the different age groups, children with a wide range of disabilities are served in public schools. Depending on the school assignment, your caseload could include children who have a single articulation error to those with multiple errors resulting in unintelligible speech. You will work with many children exhibiting speech and language disorders of unknown etiologies. You might also work with students with multiple physical and sensory disabilities. Children who have speech or language disorders associated with traumatic brain injury, cerebral palsy, emotional disorders, cognitive handicaps, hearing impairment, or cleft palate are also served in public schools.

In addition to mandating age requirements, P.L. 94-142 outlined the scope of speech-language pathology services in the public schools. The speech-language pathologist is responsible for providing the following services.

1. Identification of students with speech or language disorders through such activities as whole class or individual screenings.
2. Assessment of speech and language.
3. Speech and language treatment for students with identified communicative disorders.
4. Consultation with parents, teachers, and others regarding communicative disorders.
5. Referral to other professionals for service necessary for the remediation of a communicative disorder (Dublinske & Healey, 1978).

Though basic diagnostic and treatment principles do not vary from those appropriate in other clinical settings, several procedures may be unique to the school setting. For example, your previous experience in working with children may have followed only the clinical model; school-based speech services may be provided through different service delivery models. You may provide both direct and indirect services.

Direct services may be provided by following the traditional clinical format in which the clinician works with individual children or children in small groups. In this model, children are served in the speech-language pathologist's office or a clinical room set aside for this purpose. Students generally attend treatment sessions two times per week. Treatment may include stimulus material unrelated to classroom curriculum; however, more and more school curriculum is being incorporated into treatment when it is appropriate to the student's speech or language needs. This model commonly is referred to as the "pull-out" model because students are taken out of their classes to receive speech-language services.

You also may provide direct speech-language services in the student's class on a one to one or small group basis. In this case, you may provide treatment for one or more students in a separate area of the classroom while the rest of the class continues other activities. When classroom instruction is divided into "learning stations," you may treat children at one of the stations. The classroom teacher and aide may be responsible for two other learning stations and another station may be for independent study. Students rotate from one station to the next, typically spending 10 to 15 minutes at each station. This type of scheduling is not unusual in kindergarten and special day classes.

Speech-language services are also provided by **whole class** instruction, often in collaboration with the classroom teacher. In this model, you might present language lessons to all the students in the class. During the lesson, you also work on the speech and language objectives of the students actually enrolled on your caseload. Occasionally, you may teach a subject, such as math, to demonstrate to the teacher how changing the language in a lesson can benefit children with language disorders.

In the whole class collaborative model, the speech-language pathologist and classroom teacher discuss the needs of the class and the specific needs of the students enrolled for speech or language services. The speech-language pathologist routinely provides instruction to the whole class. A rationale for this model is that the classroom teacher will learn more effective methods of teaching the student with communicative disorders by observing the speech-language pathologist's work. Another rationale is that students will receive services in a natural communicative setting that emphasizes classroom curriculum.

A different type of whole class model of intervention is used more commonly at the secondary level. In this model, the school speech-language pathologist teaches one period of the day and students attend the class as they would their math or history classes. This may be a "language laboratory" or a language and speech class. In some schools, this class may fulfill the students' requirements for English language.

Indirect services are provided under the consultative model in which the speech-language pathologist works with the student's parents, teachers, or other professionals to address the needs of the student. In this model, the speech-language pathologist is a consultant but does not directly treat the child. For example, you may determine that a student with a language disorder no longer requires direct services. You discuss with the teacher and parents ways to modify communication to maximize the student's performance. The student remains on your caseload for a few months, and you monitor the student's progress and suggest changes.

All of these models have a place in the delivery of speech-language pathology services. However, each should be viewed on a continuum of need. Some students require intensive, direct services. Other students require less direct intervention and benefit from modification of teaching strategies. You must view each student's needs separately. Your public school practicum is an opportunity to learn when and how to effectively implement the various service delivery models.

At the university speech and hearing clinic, you may be used to working with two to three clients per term. In your school practicum, it is likely that you will be asked to gradually assume a caseload of a full-time clinician. The actual number of children on a public school clinician's caseload varies from state to state. You will usually see each student at least once a week. ASHA has recommended caseload sizes for all the speech-language services offered in the schools, with suggested caseload sizes ranging from 15 to 40 students (ASHA Committee on Language, Speech, & Hearing Services in the Schools, 1984). Unfortunately, very few, if any, school speech-language pathologists have caseloads at or below ASHA's recommended size. A reduced and manageable caseload size is a goal that is yet to be realized in the nation's public schools.

Another new experience you may have in public schools is the group treatment sessions. Due to the large number of students, public school speech-language pathologists typically serve students in small groups. Often, the number in each group depends on the total case load of the clinician. The larger the case load, the bigger the group size.

The eligibility criteria for public school students to receive speech-language pathology services differs from the criteria used in most university clinics. There are both federal and state eligibility guidelines regulating admission to the school speech-language program. These guidelines do not always coincide with the commonly accepted practices in speech-language pathology. For example, in California, a child who has only a single articulation error may not be eligible to receive services through the public school until 7 or 8 years of age (California State Department of Education, 1989). Whereas, the same child might receive treatment at a much younger age at the university clinic.

You also will learn new terminology in your school practicum. Appendix A contains a list of acronyms and abbreviations used frequently in the educational setting.

In addition to providing assessment and remediation services, school speech-language pathologists have many administrative duties. You will learn to organize and maintain records for all of the students on your caseload. You will schedule and conduct meetings with parents and other professionals.

You also will learn to work cooperatively with a variety of other professionals, including nurses, physicians, audiologists, social workers, psychologists, principals, and special and regular education teachers. You also may be called to provide staff and parent inservices.

The prerequisites to internship in the public school depend on university and state credential requirements. To begin your public school practicum, it is not necessary for you to have had experience working with groups. However, you will have completed course work relative to childhood speech and language disorders, and you will have worked with children of different ages and disorders.

Hospitals

Hospital speech-language pathology covers a wide gamut of services. When completing a clinical practicum in a hospital setting, you may work with patients in the acute care phase, inpatient rehabilitation units, outpatient departments, or at the home of the patient under the home health care. The activities of your practicum will depend both on the organization of the hospital and the requirements of your individual practicum assignment.

The speech-language pathologist providing services in the acute care setting is responsible for the speech and language evaluation and treatment of patients with many medical conditions. You will encounter patients with neurological diseases and traumatic brain injury, patients recovering from a cerebrovascular accident (CVA), and patients facing or recovering from a laryngectomy. Evaluation and treatment of dysphagia (swallowing disorders) is frequently the responsibility of the speech-language pathologist, although other professionals, notably occupational and physical therapists, also may be involved. More frequently in the rehabilitation or outpatient setting than in the acute care setting, the speech-language pathologist also may be involved in assessing and training utilization of augmentative communication equipment.

Counseling the hospital patient and the patient's family relative to the communicative disorder is a major responsibility of speech-language pathologists. Through counseling and consultation, the speech-language pathologist educates the family and the patient about the communicative disorder and assists them in learning to deal with the disorder during the rehabilitation process.

To meet the needs of the patient and the patient's family, the speech-language pathologist also must consult or work closely with numerous health care professionals. These professionals include nurses, physical therapists, occupational therapists, psychologists, audiologists, social workers, physicians, and physiatrist (physician in charge of a patient's rehabilitation). The roles of these professionals are discussed in chapter 5.

In most hospital and rehabilitation facilities, patients of all ages may be served. An exception is a pediatric setting in which you will be working exclusively with children.

As a student intern, you gradually will assume the responsibilities of the staff speech-language pathologist under the supervision of an appropriately licensed and certified speech-language pathologist on the hospital staff. The staff clinician who supervises in a hospital must follow the ASHA guidelines. A minimum of 25% of treatment sessions and a minimum of 50% of diagnostic sessions must be supervised.

Ideally, before you begin your clinical practicum at a hospital, you will have completed academic courses in aphasia, voice, and neurological disorders. You will have refreshed your knowledge of anatomy and physiology of speech and hearing mechanisms. You also will have had some experience in assessing and treating clients with communicative disorders associated with medical conditions.

A unique aspect of a hospital practicum is that you will learn to work as a member of a multidisciplinary team. To deliver the best care for your patients, you will work with other professionals such as physical therapists, nurses, occupational therapists, and physicians. The assessment and treatment decisions you make are likely to involve other team members. You will participate in "rounds" and learn how each team member contributes to the overall care and habilitation of the patient. In hospital rounds, you and other care providers go with the physician in charge to the patients' rooms. The physician may give information about the patient or ask questions about the results of the various assessments and treatments.

Unlike treatment in the public schools, individual treatment sessions are the most frequent in hospital settings. An exception might be some group language sessions. The clinician typically works with a patient in his or her office or individual treatment rooms. However, bedside evaluation and treatment are sometimes provided for patients with more acute medical conditions. For example, the patient just recovering from a stroke may not be medically stable enough to leave his or her hospital room. However, it may still be necessary for you to perform an assessment to determine the patient's current communicative status and need for intervention.

Hospitalized patients may receive speech and language services 4 or 5 days per week. Outpatients are usually seen less frequently and may be seen in the office or as part of home health services.

Hospital patients may be seen more frequently than those attending university clinics, but they may receive services for a shorter duration. Because of health care costs, most hospitals discharge patients as soon as possible, with due regard to the patient's well-being. Consequently, you may feel that you are just beginning to know the patient or observe patient progress when the patient is discharged from the hospital.

The speech-language pathology department is an integral part of the hospital's rehabilitation services. A speech-language pathologist serves as a member of a multidisciplinary team and provides assessment and intervention for patients admitted for rehabilitation services. Some patients are transferred to the rehabilitation department after discharge from the acute care setting. Other patients are discharged from the hospital for convalescence and may later be readmitted when they become candidates for rehabilitation.

In a hospital rehabilitation setting, you may have the opportunity to work with patients over a longer period of time than most of the patients in acute care settings. You will establish both short-term and long-range communicative objectives for your patients and help them to regain their independent living skills.

Individuals are sometimes discharged from the hospital acute care or rehabilitation setting before they have completed their speech or language treatment. These individuals may be served in the hospital outpatient setting or in their homes via home health services. Patients who are too ill to travel to the clinic outpatient facilities are seen in their homes.

Home health service may be provided to individuals after they are discharged from the hospital. The speech-language pathologist is one of several home care providers including nurses, physical therapists, and occupational therapists. As a home care provider, you may travel extensively because assessment and treatment are provided in patients' homes. Service delivery in the home enables you to evaluate patients' functional communication skills within their natural environments. In the homes, you also can assess the interactional patterns between the patient and his or her family.

Treatment may be enhanced by working with the patient and his or her family in their home, but there are several factors you must consider. Because you are working in an individual's home, you must be aware of cultural or traditional characteristics of the home. For example, members of a family may remove their shoes before entering the home; other families do not readily accept strangers into their homes. You also must be aware of safety factors such as the type of neighborhood a home is located in (e.g., high crime area), the presence of an aggressive and unfriendly dog in the home, the possibility of substance abuse in the home, and the overall safety of the home. Also, while in a patient's home, you cannot readily consult with other professionals.

The hospital clinician may be assigned a rotating schedule that includes home health services. For example, the clinician may work 4 months in the hospital, 4 months with home health, and 4 months with outpatients. In addition to hospital based clinicians, in-home speech services may be provided by private agencies or individual speech-language pathologists contracting for these services.

As you will find in all your practicum assignments, the speech-language pathologist in the hospital is responsible for carefully documenting assessment results, treatment plans, and patient progress. Your supervisor will assist you with the specific requirements at your hospital practicum site.

One of the frequently utilized means of communication among professionals in hospitals is through notations in the patients' charts. When reading your patients' charts, you will encounter many abbreviations, symbols, and acronyms with which you may be unfamiliar. Some of the commonly used medical abbreviations and symbols are listed in Appendix B.

This is only an overview of some of the experiences you may gain in the hospital setting. In a comprehensive medical setting, you will encounter a wide range of stimulating and challenging learning opportunities.

Skilled Nursing Facilities

Skilled nursing facilities (SNF) are designed to provide services for individuals requiring convalescent care for many medical reasons. These services are provided following discharge from the hospital and before the patients return home. The SNF also provides services for individuals who need long-term medical care. Generally, patient services in the SNF are similar to those in a hospital.

Skilled nursing care involves regularly monitoring the patient's vital signs (such as temperature, pulse, respiration), giving medications, and other types of medical care. These patients also may receive services from such other professionals as a physical therapist, speech-language pathologist, occupational therapist, recreational therapist, and social worker.

In a SNF, student clinicians work primarily with elderly patients. The communicative disorders of the patients you may work with often are associated with cerebrovascular accidents, head injury, carcinomas of the head and neck, and a variety of neurological diseases.

Speech-language pathology services in a SNF include not only assessment and treatment of communicative disorders, but also of dysphagia (swallowing disorders). Individual treatment sessions are common, though some group sessions may be held. Group sessions are helpful in promoting social communication skills in an environment where social interactions sometimes are limited. In a SNF, you will soon find that many patients fatigue quickly, and the length of both the evaluation and treatment sessions depend on the patients' health.

In addition to direct patient contact, the speech-language pathologist provides indirect services through consultation with the SNF staff. A significant part of this indirect service is to educate the staff (nurses and aides) regarding communicative disorders. Following are several goals for training the SNF staff.

1. **Train the staff to help identify patients with communicative disorders.** You will not be able to see all the patients in the facility as they are admitted. A staff well-informed about communicative problems can help you in locating individuals who need your services. In addition, such a staff will not waste your time by making many inappropriate referrals.
2. **Train the staff on ways to speak with individuals with communicative disorders.** The staff can assist with your generalization and maintenance program during their everyday interactions with your patients. More effective communication between the staff and the patients also can enhance the quality of medical care the patients receive.
3. **Train the staff to identify and change environmental factors that affect communication.** For instance, you simply may need to explain to the staff that appropriate lighting can help the hard-of-hearing individual understand speech better. You can ask the staff to prompt their patients to request before giving them something. There is much noise and activity in the SNF that can disrupt communication. Look around and make a list of suggestions to discuss with the staff.

As in other medical practicum settings, it would be ideal for you to have completed courses in aphasia, voice, and neurological disorders before beginning practicum in a SNF. A course in gerontology is highly desirable.

Rehabilitation Facilities

Rehabilitation facilities provide comprehensive services to the individual disabled by an accident or illness. The goal of rehabilitation is to maximize the individual's recovery and minimize any residual dysfunction. To derive the greatest benefit from your practicum experience in a rehabilitation facility, you should have completed course work in aphasia, neurological disorders, and voice.

Rehabilitation facilities may be a part of community hospital services or a private agency. There also are an increasing number of rehabilitation hospitals that specialize in treating the disabled. Both inpatient and outpatient services are provided by the members of a multidisciplinary team.

The rehabilitation team often includes a physiatrist, physical therapist, speech-language pathologist, occupational therapist, nurse, neuropsychologist, and social worker. There is close communication among team members whose services are interrelated. For example, based on information obtained during patient staffings, the speech-language pathologist may find that a specific patient cannot reach across midline. During speech therapy, the clinician will be careful to place pictures the patient is required to point to within the patient's reach. In another instance, the physical therapist consults with the speech-language pathologist and discovers that a patient who has been nonverbal during physical therapy sessions is able to produce single word utterances; consequently, the physical therapist prompts the patient to respond to questions verbally during treatment sessions.

The rehabilitation team also works closely with the patient's family. The family members take an active part in rehabilitating the patient. A psychologist or social worker may counsel the family members to help them deal with the emotional adjustments required. The speech-language pathologist also counsels the family members and works with them to reestablish the patient's communicative skills.

A large percentage of the population served in the rehabilitation facility include patients who have suffered head injuries resulting from automobile or motorcycle accidents. Head injuries may be called traumatic brain injury (TBI), closed head injury (CHI), or acquired brain injury (ABI). Speech and language disorders of this population include apraxia, dysarthria, and aphasia. It is not unusual for speech-language pathologists also to have patients with dysphagia or thought disorders on their caseload.

Patients recovering from cerebrovascular accidents (CVA) with associated speech and language disorders also are seen in rehabilitation facilities. Patients recovering from a CVA also may exhibit aphasia, apraxia, dysarthria, dysphagia, and cognitive disorders.

In addition to providing services for individuals recovering from head injury or stroke, some rehabilitation facilities serve individuals with orthopedic handicaps. For example, children with cerebral palsy benefit from several rehabilitative services including physical therapy, speech and language treatment, and vocational therapy.

Although the speech-language services offered in acute care hospital settings have short-term goals, those offered in rehabilitation facilities have long-range goals. The speech-language pathologist participates in ongoing evaluation and treatment of patients and assists them in obtaining long-range communicative goals. Patients served in rehabilitation facilities receive intensive treatment, sometimes two times per day, 5 to 6 days per week. Planning and preparing for these frequent treatment sessions may be another new experience for you.

The clinician may be involved in assisting the patient with relearning daily living activities and functional communication and memory skills. The clinician also may teach the use of assistive communicative devices to patients with poor prognosis for verbal communication.

The speech-language pathologist is an important member of the rehabilitation team. You will find participating in practicum at a rehabilitation site an interesting and rewarding learning experience.

Psychiatric Hospitals

Most psychiatric facilities are state operated and designed to serve individuals who are mentally ill or developmentally disabled (mentally retarded). Most of these facilities offer speech and hearing services. Although residential care is part of the psychiatric hospital, outpatient services also are available. In recent years, there has been an increased emphasis on mainstreaming the mentally ill and the developmentally disabled.

In psychiatric facilities, the speech-language pathologist provides services to both children and adults. In addition to working with individuals with speech or language disorders, the clinician may work with patients who have behavioral disorders as well. Frequently, the speech-language pathologist is requested to evaluate a patient's communicative disorder that might be contributing to his or her problem behavior. Again, the speech-language pathologist often works as a member of a multidisciplinary team, which may consist of a psychiatric nurse, a psychologist, a social worker, a psychiatrist, and other professionals.

Because of the attempts to integrate individuals who are mentally ill or developmentally disabled back into their communities, clinicians may see them in different settings. You may work in more or less restrictive facilities including state psychiatric hospitals, outpatient clinics, or schools.

The frequency and length of treatment sessions will vary depending on the needs of the patient, the specific setting the patient is seen in, and the financial resources of the patient and the agency. The length of the session is also dependent on the amount of time the patient can effectively be involved in treatment. Some of the psychiatric patients benefit from a 45-minute treatment session, whereas other patients may need a shorter session because of their limited attention span.

Clinical practicum in a psychiatric setting offers you an opportunity to work with some unique cases. You will interact with many different professionals. You will learn to work as a member of an multidisciplinary team, to resolve many behavioral issues, and to evaluate and treat individuals with communicative disorders associated with mental illness, developmental disability, or both.

Preschool Agencies

Preschool programs typically serve children ages 3 to 5 years. However, preschools now are expanding to include infants and toddlers. Although many preschools are privately operated, the primary agencies offering the services of a speech-language pathologist are government programs such as Head Start, state preschools, economic opportunity programs, and local school districts.

Since the passage of P.L. 94-142 and the later amendment of P.L. 99-457, public schools are providing many preschool services for the child with special needs. In many communities, clinicians providing speech and language services to the preschool child in the public school setting are employees of the school district. In other communities, usually due to limited resources, either financial or personnel, the school district contracts with a private practice to provide mandated services for preschool children with speech-language disorders.

In public schools and Head Start programs, the speech-language pathologist most frequently works as an **itinerant clinician** who travels from one location to another. The population served at each preschool setting is relatively small. Consequently, you will find that the itinerant speech-language pathologist providing services to these sites travels extensively, sometimes going to two or more sites per day.

Preschool programs serve children who are severely handicapped to nondisabled . The more severe the physical and sensory disabilities of the children, the greater the communicative problems exhibited by them. With children who are severely disabled , you will see the entire range of communicative disorders. To work in a preschool setting, you should have a good understanding of normal and disordered speech and language development, infant speech perception and production, and techniques of early intervention.

You also will have the opportunity to work with several service delivery models practiced in preschools. Preschool children are served individually or in small groups. Children with disorders of articulation, voice, or fluency are usually seen individually. Children with disorders of language are seen individually or in small groups. The trend in preschools is to serve children with language disorders in group settings. Often, language activities may be integrated with other social and educational activities. This will enable the child to experience more natural communicative interactions. Such integrated activities may promote generalization and maintenance.

In preschools, you will learn to provide consultative services for the child's parents and teachers. Working with the parents of preschool children may be one of the more difficult tasks of clinical practicum in the preschool setting. You may or may not have been exposed to this task in your student practicum at the university. Therefore, at the beginning of your clinical practicum at a preschool, discuss with your site supervisor your strengths and limitations in working with parents of preschool clients.

Private Clinics

Across the nation, private practices in speech-language pathology are rapidly growing. You might think that private practitioners provide speech-language pathology services only in their office to clients in individual treatment sessions. However, this scenario is only a small part of the picture. Besides working with clients in their offices, private practitioners may contract to provide speech-language pathology services for other private agencies. For example, private practitioners may serve skilled nursing facilities, home health care agencies, hospitals without speech and hearing departments, psychiatric facilities, and private preschools. They also may have contracted to serve children in local public schools.

Some private clinics may specialize. For example, one private practice may specialize in pediatric services, while another may serve adults only. Yet another private clinic may have expertise in treating patients with laryngectomy. There also are extensive private practices that hire large numbers of speech-language pathologists who contract to offer services to patients in skilled nursing facilities and home health care agencies.

Because the private practitioner is dependent on favorable public relations, you will need to have, or quickly develop, good interpersonal skills. You will not only develop your skills in assessing and treating communicative disorders, but also will gain insight into the business aspects of your profession. You will learn about marketing your services to the public and getting reimbursed by insurance companies and such governmental programs as Medicare.

Your opportunities to work with clients in private clinics may be somewhat limited because most expect and request services from an experienced, licensed, and certified professional regardless of the amount of supervision available for a student clinician. Still, there are many opportunities for working under the supervision of the speech-language pathologist providing contractual service to other agencies. Also, the speech-language pathologist with sufficient staff resources may be able to provide additional services through a student clinician for a client who needs more frequent treatment, but cannot afford it.

Students planning a practicum assignment in a private practice need a broad educational background. Clients may range from infants to elderly individuals. The entire range of communicative disorders may be treated in private settings.

Other Clinical Settings

There are many other clinical settings available to the student clinician that have not been detailed in this chapter. Among other settings, speech-language pathology services also are provided at adult day health care centers, veterans administration hospitals, and public and private clinics. The range of settings in which you might complete your clinical practicum may be limited by demographics and the university's resources. More frequently, however, the range is limited only by your own initiative. If you wish to gain practicum experience in a new setting, discuss your interest with your supervisor, clinical director, or academic advisor.

Clinical Internships

Clinical internships may be part-time or full-time. Though a part of clinical practicum, internships provide comprehensive, on-the-job experience for more advanced students. Also, an internship typically is completed in an off-campus clinical site. The qualifications of the student clinician and the requirements of the clinical site determine the type of internships available.

Part-time Internships

Part-time internships can be divided into two sections, intermittent and daily. Intermittent part-time internships allow you to participate in clinical practicum at a given site on a periodic basis. For example, you might receive a practicum assignment at a skilled nursing facility for 2 hours per day, 2 days per week. Other intermittent internships may allow your hours to vary from week to week. Daily part-time internships are much closer to the requirements of a full-time internship. You are assigned a clinical site for a specified number of hours and required to participate in practicum each day of the work week.

Part-time internships allow you to schedule your work and academic classes around clinical practicum. Some part-time practicum may be so limited that you will not learn much about the setting and the clients served there. However, in the early stages of clinical practicum, many student clinicians need additional time to assimilate and integrate new information and experiences. For these students, part-time internships are ideal.

Full-time Internships

Full-time internships require you to participate in a clinical practicum with the number of hours, work days, and holidays parallel to those of the clinical-site staff. If you are participating in a full-time practicum assignment at an elementary school, you might be there from 8:00 a.m. to 3:30 p.m., Mondays through Fridays for a specific number of weeks or total number of hours. If you were assigned to a hospital practicum site as a full-time intern you probably would be required to arrive at work at 8:00 a.m. and work until 5:00 p.m., Mondays through Fridays for a certain number of weeks or until you earn a specific number of clinical hours.

Full-time internships and even daily part-time internships provide a more comprehensive practicum experience than do intermittent assignments. In full-time internships, you may be able to experience more of the professional and interpersonal aspects of the assigned setting. In addition to direct patient contact, you also may be included in rounds or staffings and be more closely involved with allied professionals. You may attend, or even provide, staff development (training) inservices. A full-time internship allows you to experience the daily routines and pressures associated with a particular setting and to obtain a better understanding of the personal as well as professional requirements of the work setting. Part-time internships rarely provide you with this opportunity because you are not on-site long enough.

Because full-time internships are intensive and allow minimal time for class work, they often are reserved for student clinicians in their final term of graduate work or for summer practicum assignments. However, if you wish to take up a full-time internship sooner, discuss it with your advisor.

General Administrative Procedures

A primary goal of speech-language pathology training programs is to provide valuable practicum experience for student clinicians while offering and maintaining clinical services of high quality. Many administrative procedures are necessary to meet this goal.

Facilities and Equipment

The university must ensure that both on-site and off-site facilities are adequate and appropriate for clinical practicum. The university speech and hearing clinic should maintain a current inventory of evaluation instruments and supplies, provide a professional and safe environment in which to provide clinical services, and offer adequate supervision and guidance to students from qualified supervisors. The clinic should assure quality service to its clients.

Before placing students in off-campus practicum sites, the university clinic director evaluates them for their appropriateness. The clinic director verifies the qualifications and certification status of on-site supervisors, the types and number of clients served at the setting, and the number of clock hours students could obtain. The director may visit the facilities to ensure they are safe and adequately maintained. If you have any concerns about on-campus or off-campus facilities, discuss them with your clinic director.

Supervisor Qualifications

The department verifies supervisors' qualifications to ensure they have met accreditation and university standards. ASHA requires that clinical supervisors hold the ASHA CCC. Supervisors must effectively share information and assist students in developing clinical skills. The university clinic staff maintains and reviews supervisor records as frequently as a clinic assignment is made.

At the end of each clinical assignment, students have the opportunity to evaluate their supervisors. These evaluations are usually anonymous. In addition, the university periodically performs peer reviews. Constructive and specific feedback can help the clinical supervisor acquire more effective clinical teaching skills.

Clinic Fees

In conjunction with the university, the department faculty develops a fee scale for clinical services provided at the university speech and hearing clinic which is generally not for profit. Funds generated in fees are used to defray the costs of clinic materials, supplies, and equipment. Fees are implemented on a fixed or sliding scale and may be waived for clients unable to afford payment.

You may inform your clients about the clinic's fee schedule; but you have neither the responsibility, nor the authority, to reduce or waive fees. Clients or parents who ask questions about fees, waivers, payment plans, and so forth should be referred to the clinic office.

Scheduling Practicum Assignments

Scheduling and assignment of practicum experiences are made on the basis of the student's experience, the student's clinical clock hour needs, the student's specific area of interest, availability of practicum sites, the number of clients seeking services, and the availability of clinical supervisors. Because of these and other variables to be considered in making clinical practicum assignments, you may not always get

the kind of assignments you desire. However, the better the communication between you and the clinic director (or other individual in
charge of scheduling), the greater the likelihood of you having a
successful practicum experience. Therefore, follow the format your
university uses in registering for practicum each term and for expressing your practicum needs ahead of time.

Student Records

Prior to being admitted into clinical practicum, students' records are
reviewed to find out if they meet the academic requirements for clinical
practicum. Although ASHA provides minimum guidelines for student
performance, individual universities may have additional requirements
the students must meet.

The clinic staff maintains records of student clinicians. These
records are reviewed periodically to ensure they meet both university
and ASHA guidelines for clinical practicum, including the types of
patients served and number of clinical hours earned. It is important
that you accurately communicate, through the forms your department
uses, the clock hours you have earned and the clinical experiences you
have completed.

The training director (or the department chairman) ensures that
an evaluation of your performance is written at the end of each clinical
assignments. The supervisor discusses your evaluation with you and
places a copy of the evaluation in your file. The evaluation of your
clinical skills and the corresponding grade will influence your future
practicum assignments. If your clinical skills are weak, your continued
participation in clinical practicum may be a matter for discussion. If you
disagree with an evaluation of your practicum, you should discuss your
concerns with your supervisor. If necessary, follow established procedures students must follow to protest evaluations.

Clinic Supplies, Materials, and Equipment

The student participating in clinical practicum will use a variety of
supplies, materials, and equipment. The university clinic and many off-
campus sites provide most of these items. However, you also will be
required to purchase some materials, equipment, and supplies you use.

You will want to begin building your own inventory of materials and supplies throughout your clinical practicum regardless of the amount of materials and equipment available to you.

Clinic supplies are consumable items. These include tongue depressors, gauze, cotton swabs, gloves, finger cots, tissue, and disinfectant. Carefully follow your clinics' protocol regarding disposal of these items. Some sites designate specific containers in which to dispose supplies used in oral examinations and materials that have come in contact with saliva or blood during evaluation or treatment sessions.

Clinical materials also are categorized as consumable or expendable items. Typically included in this category are tests, test response forms, and such treatment materials as articulation cards, language programs, and books.

Your clinic library or media center may have a wide variety of tests for the evaluation of communicative disorders. Tests are generally arranged by alphabetical order or organized by the type of disorder the test is designed to evaluate. Follow the check-out procedures outlined at your university or clinical site. The same test will be used over and over again by many other individuals, so handle it carefully. Tests are expensive and the less money that has to be spent to replace worn out or lost tests, the more money that the clinic will have available to upgrade materials, equipment, and facilities.

As you progress in your clinical practicum you may want to, or be required to, take the opportunity to use many assessment instruments. Instead of continually administering the same test across clients, experiment. Learn and administer new tests. Find out which tests evaluate what they purport to evaluate, which tests are standardized for specific populations, and which speech and language behaviors might better be evaluated through analysis of speech samples. After you graduate, you will be selecting your own tests. Therefore, take time to learn to objectively evaluate most of the published tests made available to you at a practicum site.

Test response forms are also considered clinic supplies because they are consumable. Response forms are expensive, especially when they must be supplied to 20 to 40 student clinicians per semester. Use the response forms judiciously. Do not request or take more forms than you need. Some university clinics provide student clinicians with only one response form per semester for each client, and require the student to pay for any additional forms needed because of incorrect scoring or lost response form. It is not appropriate to photocopy response forms for clinical use unless the publisher specifically gives permission to reproduce the forms.

In addition to numerous tests, your clinic will have a supply of treatment materials. The type and quantity of materials differ across campuses and clinical sites. Generally available are a selection of articulation cards depicting pictures designed to evoke corresponding phonemes in a variety of word positions. Also, you frequently will have access to picture or photo decks representing many vocabulary and language concepts. Comprehensive language programs and books also may be available. Your clinic may supply different types of toys for use with younger clients. There is an abundance of commercial items available, although often the theoretical basis of the faculty and clinic staff influence the types of materials made available to the student clinician.

Treatment materials are the most individual or personalized of items used in clinical practicum. Therefore, it is not unusual for student clinicians to develop their materials. You can develop your materials by drawing pictures, using pictures from books or magazines, creating charting forms, accumulating lists of words, phrases, and sentences designed to teach phonemes or language behaviors, creating pictures using computer graphics, and developing an activity file of various treatment techniques and ideas.

Many student clinicians find it functional, as well as beneficial, to allow their clients to create some of their treatment materials. With the assistance of a parent, a young client might be asked to cut pictures out of a magazine and bring them to his or her treatment session to put into a "speech book." Another client might be asked to bring in newspaper articles to discuss during a treatment session. You may ask clients with good drawing skills to draw picture cards for use in their treatment sessions and home practice assignments.

In the school setting, clinicians increasingly are using curriculum materials as treatment materials. Clinicians in other settings may emphasize naturally occurring activities or events to evoke speech and language behaviors. Personalized materials created by the student clinician usually meet a specific need and are, consequently, functional; best of all, they are never checked out by another clinician.

Clinical equipment is nonexpendable. It is something that is used, one would hope, over a long period of time. Clinical equipment generally is much more expensive than supplies and materials. Examples of clinical equipment include audiometers, computers, tape recorders, sound level meters, auditory trainers, and augmentative communication devices. Less expensive items like flashlights, stethoscopes, dental mirrors, and therapy mirrors are also in this category.

Again, note that the longer the life of the equipment, the more your clinic can invest in new equipment rather than simply replacing lost or broken equipment. Handle the clinic equipment carefully. If you have questions about the appropriate way to utilize an instrument, ask your supervisor for assistance. Be careful when taking or returning equipment. If equipment is broken or parts missing when you check it out, notify the clinic secretary or your supervisor so that the equipment can be repaired. When you return equipment, make sure it is replaced correctly, and carefully, in its container or storage space.

In this age of rapidly advancing technology, there is an ever increasing amount of equipment available for the speech-language pathologist. Some of the equipment is priced within the budget of the student clinician, and you may want to purchase a few items to add to your personal inventory. When deciding on the purchase of a piece of equipment, determine if the equipment is something that you will use frequently, or if it is something for which there is no substitute. For example, a flashlight is inexpensive, you will use it frequently, and there really is not a better substitute for it. An audiometer, however, is expensive, you may or may not use it regularly, but there is not a substitute for it unless referrals for audiological testing are easily made. On the other hand, an augmentative communication device may be used for a single client, is generally expensive, and, rather than carrying an inventory of augmentative equipment, the client may be referred to a clinic specializing in augmentative communication.

The supplies, materials, and equipment that you need often are dependent on your clinical practicum site. It is to your advantage to experience a variety of materials and equipment in many different clinical settings.

Now that you know some of the different clinical sites and practicum experiences available, you can begin planning your clinical program with your advisor. The clinical practicum portion of your training may be important in deciding on the setting in which you want to work after graduation.

3

The Conduct of the Student Clinician

Training in speech-language pathology includes the acquisition of knowledge about communication and its disorders and skills in assessing and treating those disorders. However, an equally important part of training is not discussed formally in most textbooks or classes. This part is the acquisition of certain behavior patterns considered professionally appropriate. Professional behavior and the various codes and regulations governing this behavior will be discussed in this chapter.

General Professional Behavior

Throughout their enrollment in clinical practicum, student clinicians will have many opportunities to represent the profession of speech-language pathology, the university department and its clinic, and the university at large. Student clinicians interact with numerous clients, care providers, professionals, and related agencies in the community. Therefore, student clinicians must acquire appropriate and acceptable professional behavior.

49

In addition to the Code of Ethics of the American Speech-Language-Hearing Association (ASHA), general rules of professional behavior include punctuality in meeting clinical appointments and clinic deadlines, working cooperatively with office staff, supervisors, and other student clinicians, assuming responsibility for clinic equipment and clinic facilities, being well prepared for each clinical session, and maintaining appropriate dress and demeanor. Professional demeanor is one of the initial factors on which a student clinician is evaluated.

In the university clinic, the student clinician often is the first person to contact a client. The student clinician's initial meeting with the client sets the stage for future clinical relationships and may influence the client's willingness to pursue treatment. It is important for the client to see the clinician as a self-confident and well-trained person. The client must think that the student clinician is capable of providing quality clinical services.

At off-campus practicum sites, the student clinician is a representative of the university. Based on an individual student's professional behavior or lack of it, a practicum site may continue to offer or withdraw its offer to provide practicum experiences for other student clinicians. Although student clinicians beginning off-campus practicum should be as well prepared for the assignment as possible, no student is expected to know all procedures and regulations of the site. However, each student is expected to perform adequately and professionally. You should meet the deadlines, maintain regular attendance, work cooperatively with the site staff, learn new procedures, and follow the guidelines related to clinical practicum in a particular setting.

Even if you do not know some of the special rules and regulations of the off-campus site where you will complete your clinical internship, you should know the ASHA Code of Ethics. You will have studied these codes before starting your clinical practicum at the university clinic, but it may be a good idea to reread them before you start your internship in an off-campus site.

ASHA Code of Ethics

The ASHA Code of Ethics gives guidelines of professional behavior for individuals providing clinical services in speech-language pathology or audiology. There is no legal basis for enforcement of the Code of Ethics except in states that have adopted the code as part of licensure requirements. However, a professional violating the code of ethics may lose his or her ASHA certification, membership in ASHA, or both.

The interpretation, administration, and enforcement of the Code of Ethics is the responsibility of the **Ethical Practices Board (EPB)** of ASHA. In order to maintain ASHA certification, ASHA members are required to uphold and abide by the Code of Ethics. Many employers require that their employees providing speech-language pathology services hold current ASHA certification. Consequently, the Code of Ethics and the EPB have a significant impact on the profession.

The ASHA Code of Ethics is comprised of **principles of ethical conduct, proscriptions of conduct**, and **matters of professional propriety** (ASHA Council on Professional Ethics, 1991). A proposed revision of the Code of Ethics reorganizes the principles, and eliminates the proscriptions and matters of professional propriety (ASHA Council on Professional Ethics, 1991). The proposed revision includes four principles of ethics with specific rules of ethics outlined under the heading of individual principles. The intent of the Code of Ethics— to provide an outline for the preservation of high professional standards—remains unchanged. Following are the five major principles of the Code.

1. Individuals shall hold paramount the welfare of persons served professionally.
2. Individuals shall maintain high standards of professional competence.
3. Individuals' statements to persons served professionally and to the public shall provide accurate information about the nature and management of communicative disorders and about the profession and services rendered by its practitioners.
4. Individuals shall honor their responsibilities to the public, their profession, and their relationships with colleagues and members of allied professions.
5. Individuals shall uphold the dignity of the profession and freely accept the profession's self-imposed standards (ASHA Council on Professional Ethics, 1991).

All students participating in clinical practicum are required to comply with the ASHA Code of Ethics. The Code helps you in developing ethically responsible professional behaviors. The information outlined in the Code of Ethics not only helps you answer questions related to professional and clinical issues, but also to understand the rationale for certain clinic procedures.

The entire Code, as well as revisions, are published periodically in the *Asha* magazine. The following discussion emphasizes specific areas of the Code; however, you should read and understand the complete Code of Ethics. Appendix C contains a copy of the Code of Ethics revised in January 1991.

The Client Welfare

Principle I of the Code of Ethics is straightforward and not easily misinterpreted: "Individuals shall hold paramount the welfare of persons served professionally." The difficult part for beginning student clinicians, however, is determining what is best for the person being served. If you have a question about the legitimacy or efficacy of a particular evaluation or treatment procedure, discuss it in advance with your clinical supervisor. The Code mandates that services be evaluated to determine their effectiveness and that adequate records be maintained.

Treatment Efficacy. The Code of Ethics continues to address treatment efficacy by stating that treatment should not be provided to clients who may not be expected to benefit from treatment. The Code also prohibits continuing unnecessary treatment. Again, these are two issues that often are difficult for student clinicians to resolve. First, professionals and agencies sometimes disagree regarding these issues. For example, a speech-language pathologist may judge that a patient with brain injury could benefit from speech-language services. However, the insurance company may not approve payment for those services because, in the judgment of the company, the patient would not benefit from treatment. In this instance, the clinician may feel frustrated that he or she cannot provide needed service, but he or she has not acted unethically in recommending treatment.

Unfortunately, economics governs the administration of private businesses and the business that holds little regard for ethical practice may attempt to put the speech-language pathologist in a compromising position. For example, a speech-language pathologist may be instructed to provide services for a specific number of patients per day. If there are not sufficient numbers of appropriate patients, the clinician may be pressured to increase his or her caseload by enrolling patients for whom the benefit of treatment is questionable. Clinicians who enroll patients in treatment because of such pressures when they are reasonably sure that the patient would not benefit from treatment (e.g., because of the patient's extremely poor health) will have violated the Code of Ethics and will have acted unethically.

Second, professionals themselves may disagree on who benefits from treatment and for how long. For example, two speech-language pathologists may not agree on the appropriate chronological age for treatment of a specific communicative disorder. Also, progress of some individuals (for instance, a person with a severe cognitive impairment) may be extremely slow and efficacy of treatment difficult to assess. Clinicians who maintain objective and accurate records of client behaviors will be better able to judge the efficacy of individual treatment than those who rely on subjective judgment and memory to evaluate client progress.

Is it considered unethical to not record all client responses? No. However, failure to maintain adequate records could be construed as unethical. Your records should document changes or lack of changes in the target behaviors over treatment sessions. Continuing the same treatment when repeated measures show no change in the client behaviors is certainly unethical. Do you necessarily have to dismiss the client? No. But you certainly should change the treatment procedure.

There is no single formula to determine which individuals can benefit from treatment or when treatment should be discontinued. Social, educational, psychological, and health factors affect your decision. You should evaluate your clients and attempt to make the appropriate determination, but you should never try to enroll or dismiss a client without first discussing the matter with your clinical supervisor.

Informed Consent. The Code covers several rules on providing information to clients. Basically, the clients must be given enough information so they can make an informed decision to continue treatment or not. This decision is informed consent. Individuals must be given information related to possible consequences of treatment and no treatment.

University clinics do not, as a rule, require individuals refusing treatment to sign a written statement verifying their refusal of treatment and their understanding of possible consequences of that refusal. However, many clinics frequently require clients to initial or sign a plan of treatment to confirm their knowledge of the proposed services. If clients are not required to submit a written acknowledgment of the treatment plan, you should note in the records when the plan was discussed with the client and the client's apparent understanding of the discussion (Flower, 1984). Each off-campus site will have its guidelines for obtaining client consent that student clinicians should follow.

Principle I directs that clients be informed fully regarding the nature and possible effects of the service. This principle gives guidelines for providing prognostic information. Beginning clinicians sometimes do not know how to reply to clients who ask if a specific treatment will "cure" them, or even how a specific procedure will affect their communicative disorder. Principle I forbids clinicians to guarantee treatment results. However, you can make an informed, reasonable, prognostic statement. For example, you should not say, "After 6 weeks of treatment, you will no longer stutter." However, you may say, "This type of treatment has been successful with many individuals who exhibited problems similar to yours. Based on the diagnostic information I have and what I think is your level of motivation for change, the chances of improvement in your speech fluency are good." Ethically justified prognostic statements are those that are probabilistic statements based on valid and reliable information about the client and the accumulated scientific evidence in the discipline. Therefore, prognostic statements should not be made without first ensuring that all necessary information has been obtained and is accurate. You must discuss your client's prognosis with your clinical supervisor before you report it to the client.

Informed consent also requires that clients be told if the treatment they receive is part of a research program. The clients must be informed clearly of the nature of research and the possible effects. The clients must be given a free choice to participate in the treatment research or opt for other kinds of treatment programs. The clients who agree to participate in an experimental treatment program retain their right to withdraw from it at any time and without prejudice.

In the university clinic, as well as at off-campus sites, it is explained clearly to the client that student clinicians provide services under the supervision of a certified professional. You must never misrepresent your status to the public.

Before providing services, you should check to ensure that all consent forms are signed by your clients. Each site will have different forms. Check with your clinical supervisor if you are not sure what forms are used at your site.

Confidentiality. One of the ethical proscriptions under Principle I states that, "Individuals must not reveal to unauthorized persons any professional or personal information obtained from the person served professionally, unless required by law or unless necessary to protect the welfare of the person or the community." In addition, legal protection of the client's right to privacy is provided by federal and state laws.

Client confidentiality is a recurring theme at university clinics. There are two reasons for this. First, much of the learning at the university level occurs by individuals sharing information and experiences with each other. Second, persons not directly involved with treatment may observe the clients receiving services.

Because students frequently discuss their clients with each other, client confidentiality may be violated easily. Observers not directly involved with service delivery may discuss clients in such a way as to violate the client confidentiality. You need to be aware of your client's right to confidentiality and monitor both your written and verbal communications to ensure those rights. The following are guidelines to help ensure client confidentiality.

1. Do not discuss your client by name except with your clinical supervisor, clinic staff, or as necessary during clinical meetings.
2. Do not discuss your client in public areas.
3. If you present information about your client during a class assignment, do not refer to your client by name. You can easily refer to your client as "my client."
4. Do not leave reports, lesson plans, or other written information containing client information unattended.
5. Follow all the office rules regarding checking out and returning client folders and reports.
6. Do not take client folders home and do not remove information from them.
7. Do not discuss your client with other professionals or persons in other agencies unless your client has approved the communication, or unless your supervisor has approved the communication in order to protect the welfare of the client or the community.
8. Remind your observers that they should respect client confidentiality.
9. Comply with all clinic rules regarding release of information to other agencies or individuals.

The very nature of university training programs requires some relaxation of the rule of client confidentiality. Students constantly observe assessment and treatment sessions. Consequently, the clinical services offered to individuals through the university training programs are less confidential than those that are offered in private clinics. This is acceptable so long as the client has given informed consent for being observed.

Written consent must be obtained also for any photographs or videotapes used in the training program. A separate consent should be obtained for any photographs or videotapes used for public viewing, such as at a health fair or community education program.

Flower (1984) discusses three types of consent related to disclosure of confidential information: implied consent, written consent, and consent inherent in the private interests of the client. **Implied consent** means that individuals seeking services implicitly approve access to their records by staff or support personnel without the need for written authorization. For example, it is not necessary for the clinic secretary to obtain written authorization before accessing a client's record because reviewing client records is typically a part of a secretary's duties.

Release of information to individuals or agencies outside of the facility requires a written authorization or **written consent**. The clinic secretary at your university clinic or at an off-campus practicum site can give you information on the consent form required and the procedures for completing it.

Consent inherent in the private interests of the client is assumed when release of information is considered to be in the best interest of the client. This form of consent generally occurs between the professional and members of the client's family. Again, without first discussing a specific situation with a clinical supervisor, student clinicians should treat all client information as confidential. This precaution will allow you to avoid the need to justify disclosure of confidential information.

Discrimination: To "hold paramount the welfare of the individuals served professionally," the Code prohibits discrimination. Decisions related to delivery of service must not be based on "race, sex, age, religion, national origin, sexual orientation, or handicapping condition." Student clinicians provide speech-language pathology services for a wide variety of individuals. Obviously, there will be certain persons you enjoy working with more than others. It is important to remember that clinical judgments and recommendations must be made on clinical data and not on unrelated factors.

Professional Qualifications

The Code of Ethics also defines the professional qualifications of individuals providing speech-language pathology services. According to Principle II, "Individuals shall maintain high standards of professional competence." Individuals providing independent speech-language pathology services, or supervising the delivery of those services, must hold the Certificate of Clinical Competence in Speech-Language Pathology (CCC-SLP).

Continuing Education. As you know, the CCC implies that the minimum educational and clinical qualifications have been met. The Code expands on these qualifications by addressing the need for continuing education and for sharing information with colleagues in the profession.

To maintain a high standard of professional competence, speech-language pathologists must continue their education, even after they have received their CCC. Some organizations require members to earn a certain number of continuing education "units" or "hours," to maintain their affiliation or license. While not requiring this, ASHA strongly encourages continuing education and awards a certificate of recognition to members who accumulate continuing education units.

You may have already discovered that researchers and clinicians rapidly and constantly produce new information about communicative disorders. Some of what you learned in many undergraduate classes may be outdated by the time you start your clinical practicum. You are busy keeping up with course work, but you must remain current. You can begin the practice of self-study by reading journals and recently published books in speech-language pathology. You can also attend many conferences and workshops to gain current scientific and professional information.

Preparation. The Code directs individuals to be well prepared for the services they provide and to require individuals under their supervision to be well prepared. In training programs, the student "uses" the supervisor's license and certification to learn the techniques of the profession.

You must be well prepared to work with your clients. As part of your preparation, you must acquire and organize information about normal and disordered communication, methods of assessment and treatment, various diagnostic and therapeutic materials, and all clinical procedures including the Code of Ethics.

Many speech-language pathologists could be classified as "generalists." They are clinicians well versed in the assessment and treatment of the more commonly encountered communicative disorders. However, many generalists may have limited knowledge and experience in specific disorders or treatment procedures. For this reason, a clinician may not, for example, be able to adequately serve a patient with laryngectomy or stuttering. At university clinics, student clinicians commonly are required to complete course work in a specific communicative disorder before they are assigned a client with that disorder. This policy ensures that the student clinician at least is prepared academically to work with clients who have specific disorders.

Minimally, you will have a general background in a specific disorder before you are assigned a client with that disorder. However, you may be required to do additional research to effectively serve that client. If you are unable to find the information you need, your supervisor will refer you to appropriate sources. Maintaining professional competence is a continuous process.

Referral. Related to providing only services that one is well prepared to provide is the need to "identify competent, dependable referral sources for persons served professionally." It is customary to provide several names of qualified professionals when making a referral. You should not refer clients to an individual practicing speech-language pathology or audiology without a current ASHA certification. Your practicum site will have a list of qualified professionals for referrals. Your referral list may include other speech-language pathologists, audiologists, otolaryngologists, orthodontists, dentists, and physicians.

It is important to refer to individuals who are both qualified and cooperative. If you have had difficulty obtaining necessary information from a professional, you may want to avoid referring to that individual.

As with all other major clinical decisions, you should not make a referral without first discussing the matter with your clinical supervisor. The reason for the referral and to whom the referral will be made must be approved by your clinical supervisor.

Representation to the Public

Representation of the profession to the public is addressed in Principle III of the Code of Ethics. Principle III instructs that "individuals must not misrepresent their training or competence," and that, "public statements providing information about professional services and products must not contain representations or claims that are false, deceptive or misleading." Directly related to the university training program is the need for clients to fully understand that students in the program provide services. This information is given to clients who contact the speech and hearing clinic to inquire about services available. The clients also are told about the clinic schedule and fees. Individuals who want to find other services are referred to qualified speech-language pathologists in the area.

Professional Relationships

The Code of Ethics also addresses professional relationships. The Code states that, "Individuals shall honor their responsibilities to the public, their profession, and their relationships with colleagues and members of allied professions." The Code further mandates that "Individuals should strive to increase knowledge within the profession and share research with colleagues." The Code continues to explain that, "Individuals should establish harmonious relations with colleagues and members of other professions, and endeavor to inform members of related professions of services provided by speech-language pathologists and audiologists, as well as seek information from them."

Sharing Information. Within the competitive arena of the university training program, professional relationships are sometimes difficult to establish. Students hesitate in sharing "too much" information with their fellow students thinking that they will then, somehow, fall behind those students in academic or clinical skills. Some students do not ask questions of their instructors, supervisors, or other students, because of their fear of appearing ignorant. Unfortunately, these types of behaviors interfere with optimal learning.

Ethically, some information may be shared freely and others may not be. For example, it would be unethical for a student to discuss a client by name in an open forum involving persons not related to service delivery. However, it would not be unethical, and might benefit both the students, if they shared with each other procedures, materials, or techniques that one found to be especially effective in a clinic session.

Discussing Other Clinicians. You will work with clients who have received services over a long period of time or have received services from other professionals. Some of these clients may remark that "The other clinician did things differently," or that "The other clinician did not help me at all."

Do not make judgmental statements about other clinicians or professionals. Give the client facts. Keep the focus on clinical techniques and procedures, not on other clinicians. For example, "I've had a lot of success with this procedure. In fact, research studies have shown that this procedure is effective with people with your kind of problem." You not only want to "establish harmonious relationships with colleagues," but must consider that the client may be giving you inaccurate information. If the client tells you something that suggests that some professional may have acted unethically, report it to your clinical supervisor.

Assigning Credit: The Code of Ethics directs that credit (or recognition) be proportionally given to individuals who have contributed to a written work. Your reports submitted for academic or clinical course work must contain references and credit other individuals involved in the work. For example, if you and another student collaborate in evaluating a client and writing the assessment report, both of you should sign the report. (Your supervisor must also sign the report.) If you are reporting information described in a different report, the name of that evaluator and the date of the report should be noted.

Upholding the Standards of the Profession

The final principle of the Code establishes that individuals must comply freely with the standards of the professions, in this case the standards ASHA suggests in its Code of Ethics and other guidelines. In addition to individually upholding the Code, clinicians who have a "reason to believe that a member or certificate holder may have violated the Code of Ethics," must report to the EPB (Ethical Practice Board). However, the student clinician reports such incidents to the clinical supervisor. The clinical supervisor, the clinic director, and the department chair will decide what action might be taken.

So far, we have highlighted the major sections of the Code of Ethics that student clinicians may be involved with. The Code also contains additional proscriptions and prescriptions. Read the Code of Ethics in Appendix C. Which of the following situations would you consider a violation of the Code of Ethics? What would be an ethical way to handle each situation?

1. You were busy studying for midterm exams and "just didn't have enough time" to completely prepare for your clinical session.
2. You are beginning your second year of graduate school. A speech-language pathologist in private practice telephones and asks you to work as an aide. How would you reply? Are there any specific requirements you would need to comply with to be employed as a speech aide? Could you earn clinical clock hours? Could you perform other clinical services?

3. The mother of one of your clients contacts you and asks if you would be available to tutor her child. How would you respond?
4. A clinical supervisor allows students, who were continually ill-prepared for their clinical assignments, to continue in clinical practicum.
5. You are working with a client who is also receiving speech-language services at another facility. You do not agree with the type of treatment being provided by the other speech-language pathologist. What would you do?
6. Your supervisor suggested that you use certain treatment procedures with one of your clients. You were unsure of how to implement the procedures, but could not get to school during your supervisor's office hours to discuss the procedures. You decided to work with your client anyway, because if you were doing something wrong, your supervisor would see it and come in to help you.
7. A man you have been working with for two months tells you that he just tested positive for HIV (human immunodeficiency virus) infection. He wants to continue treatment, but does not want anyone to know about his medical history except you.

Other Codes and Regulations

Reporting Suspected Child Abuse

Although students should first assume that all client information is confidential, there are specific state laws governing disclosure of information in order to protect the well-being of the client or of the public. A clear example is a clinician's responsibility to report suspected child abuse.

Based on federal laws and regulations, states have established laws regulating the reporting of suspected child abuse. The reporting requirements differ across states. The definition of child abuse, the age range of victims, and the agency to whom the suspected abuse is reported vary also from state to state. Nevertheless, suspected child abuse must be reported. In most states, the individual suspecting the abuse must report it. The individual cannot leave the reporting to the agency he or she works for (Flower, 1984).

Child abuse is not always visible or easily identified. You may have a client who comes in with human bite marks on his or her arm. This would be a fairly obvious signal for suspecting abuse. However, another child may arrive for his or her treatment with a bruised face. This might suggest abuse, or that the child fell while running. You must not jump to conclusions, but you must not disregard signs of possible child abuse.

If you suspect child abuse, inform your supervisor immediately. Each clinical site will have its reporting procedure. You should know these procedures and follow them when necessary.

Dress Code

There is not a universal dress code that student clinicians must follow in all practicum sites. However, all clinics have guidelines for what they consider appropriate professional attire. Contrary to some beliefs, you are not expected to go out and purchase an entirely new wardrobe. Typically, shorts, jeans, sandals, and strapless dresses are not considered appropriate for professional clothing. If you have a question as to whether something is appropriate to wear, do not wear it.

At off-campus practicum sites, dress may be more or less formal than at the university clinic. If no information is offered, ask your off-campus supervisor about the dress code or guidelines at the site. Occasionally, a supervisor will say that, "Anything is okay to wear," while the supervisor and the rest of the staff dresses very formally. In this case, it is best to dress as similarly to the staff as possible. In all cases, dressing with a view to appearing professional is desirable.

From being a student during certain times of the day to being a clinician at other times of the day may be a difficult transition. Professional dress helps you make that transition. It also prompts the client to regard you more as a "professional" and less as a student.

Liability Insurance

Though you are a student in training, you still provide direct client services when you engage in clinical practicum. Therefore, you may be held responsible for your actions. Clinicians may be liable for any inappropriate or negligent service that results in damage or harm to a client.

All student clinicians should have liability insurance before beginning their clinical practicum. You can obtain information from your clinic office regarding the procedures for obtaining liability insurance. In some locations, students pay for insurance directly to the university. In other locations, students are required to independently purchase insurance and then provide the proof of coverage.

Insurance typically is purchased on an annual basis. A low cost group insurance is available for students and professional practitioners. Information can be obtained at your clinic or by contacting ASHA.

To avoid any suspicion of negligence or malpractice, you must closely follow the ASHA Code of Ethics, comply with all clinic procedures, and maintain appropriate communications with your supervisor. You also should be knowledgeable in current standards of care for the disorders you treat. Periodically, ASHA publishes **Position Statements** and **Guidelines**. These documents specify ASHA's official position on controversial clinical or scientific issues, recommend appropriate courses of professional actions, and summarize state-of-the-art information on selected issues. Clinicians should keep themselves current on these position statements and guidelines.

Health Regulations

Because you will be working closely with people, you must follow certain health regulations. These regulations provide protection for you and your clients from various communicable diseases. Because you work with many different individuals, you are at a greater risk for exposure to a communicable disease, than, for instance, a computer programmer might be. Each practicum site may have different health regulations. You must follow the regulations of your clinical assignment. General health regulations include the following procedures.

1. **Rubella vaccination.** All individuals should have a rubella vaccination. It is required only one time. Rubella, also known as German Measles, is a viral disease often accompanied by a fever and a rash. Although children who have rubella rarely experience any complications, the virus can be a teratogen to a developing fetus with the possibility of intrauterine death, spontaneous abortion, or many types of congenital defects (Benenson, 1990).

2. **Mumps vaccination.** Mumps is a viral disease. It is accompanied by tenderness and swelling of one or more of thesalivary glands and fever. There is no clear evidence linking mumps during pregnancy with congenital malformations. However, because of the incidence of testicular

mumps in the male population, male health care providers are advised or required to have mumps vaccination. The frequency of mumps has decreased since early childhood immunization has become available. However, an increase in mumps was reported in the United States in both 1986 and 1987 (Benenson, 1990).

3. **Tuberculin skin test.** (PPD—Purified Protein Derivative) Tuberculosis is an infectious mycobacterial disease. Generally, it has decreased in occurrence in developed countries, but has plateaued or increased in frequency in the population of persons testing positive for HIV infection. Tuberculosis most often involves the lungs and if left untreated, can result in death or other serious complications. The initial infection to tuberculosis often is not recognized. This is one of the reasons students, in close contact with a variety of individuals in their clinical experiences, are required to have a tuberculin skin test on a regular basis. Clinics may require a skin test annually. Public schools often require the skin test less frequently because the incidence of tuberculosis is less in children and increases in the aging population (Benenson, 1990).

4. **Use of gloves.** Wear latex gloves when performing oral exams, during any invasive procedure of the oral cavity (such as dysphagia assessment or treatment), or during any contact with blood or bodily fluids with visible blood (ASHA Committee on Quality Assurance, 1990).

5. **Handwashing.** Wash your hands before and after working with a client. Handwashing is considered one of the best ways to prevent the spread of disease. In addition, avoid touching your hands to your mouth, eyes, or nose when working with your clients.

6. **Disinfect or sterilize equipment.** Follow your practicum site's procedures regarding sterilization and disinfection of equipment. Disinfection can be performed using 1:100 solution of household bleach (sodium hypochlorite) to water (ASHA Committee on Quality Assurance, 1990). Commercial disinfectant is also available. McMillan and Willette (1988) advised that environmental surfaces such as tables, tape recorders, and audiometers be disinfected prior to and following each client contact. However, more recent information suggests that "equipment not contaminated by blood or bodily fluids containing visible signs of blood need not be cleaned after each use." (ASHA Committee on Quality Assurance, 1990).

7. **Use disposable materials.** Whenever possible use disposable materials.
8. **Stay home if you are ill.** If you are ill, cancel your clinical appointments. You probably will not be very effective as a clinician anyway and may transmit your illness to your client.

For obvious reasons, the spread of AIDS/HIV infection currently is a major health concern (ASHA Committee on Quality Assurance, 1989; ASHA Committee on Quality Assurance, 1990; McMillan & Willette, 1988). AIDS (acquired immune deficiency syndrome) is considered the last clinical stage of HIV infection. Present information indicates that transmission is by sexual exposure and exposure to blood or tissue. Although progress is being reported in the drug treatment for HIV infection, there is no known treatment for the primary immune deficiency (Benenson, 1990).

Depending on the work environment, there are other diseases of which the speech-language pathologist should be aware. However, it is not the purpose of this chapter to outline all possible diseases to which one may be exposed. It is hoped that students will seriously consider the potential for exposure to communicable diseases, both the inconvenient types as well as the life-threatening ones, and closely follow all disease control procedures established at clinical practicum sites.

It is clear to you by now that you should follow many codes and regulations. Besides health regulations, students must comply with the ASHA Code of Ethics, codes and regulations of practicum sites, as well as federal and state laws. Many of the codes and regulations overlap. For instance, to protect the client's welfare, informed consent is required and confidentiality of information is mandated. However, also to protect the client's welfare, confidentiality may be breached if child abuse is suspected.

In abiding by the Code of Ethics and state and federal laws, you may occasionally encounter guidelines that could be interpreted in different ways. In all such cases, you must consider the well-being of your clients as an important basis to make decisions. Your supervisor or clinic director will be there to help you make appropriate and ethical decisions. ASHA, your state speech-language-hearing association, and your state licensure agency also are important institutions that help resolve professional questions.

4

The Supervisor and the Student Clinician

Y our clinical practicum in speech-language pathology is a three-way process involving you, your supervisor, and your client. Your supervisor is your clinical mentor. In many ways, your supervisor helps you acquire the knowledge and skills necessary to become an independent and competent clinician who can provide quality service for clients. The effectiveness of your practicum experience depends, partly, on the relationship developed between you and your supervisor. Each of you have different roles and responsibilities in the development of your clinical skills.

The Role of the Clinical Supervisor

The primary role of the clinical supervisor is to help a student learn clinical skills through clinical practicum. However, the clinical supervisor at the university clinic may wear many different hats. In addition to providing direct and indirect clinical supervision, the supervisor must assure a successful learning experience for the student clinician and quality clinical services to the client. Also, the supervisor must fulfill other managerial or academic obligations. Many university clinics

67

have a staff of full-time supervisors who do little or no classroom teaching. Many other university clinics have academic faculty members supervising clinical practicum. Supervisors also may be assigned a variety of administrative duties.

It is important that the student clinician understand some of the supervisor's responsibilities and limitations in order to avoid misunderstandings or incorrect expectations. It is equally important that the clinical supervisor be aware of the student clinician's prior experience and clearly define practicum guidelines and expectations.

What to Expect From Your Clinical Supervisor

The clinical supervisor facilitates the student clinician's practicum experience. This facilitation includes direct teaching of clinical methods, self-evaluation, clinical analysis, and problem solving skills. The ASHA report on supervision in speech-language pathology and audiology identified 13 supervisory tasks (ASHA Committee on Supervision, 1985). These tasks provide a guideline for supervision. Many of them have been integrated into the following sections providing an overview of what student clinicians can expect from their supervisors.

Develop and Maintain Effective Communication. It is important that the clinical supervisor and student clinician establish a cooperative working relationship to enhance the student's clinical practicum experience and assure the delivery of quality services. Some clinical supervisors are available before, during, and after clinic sessions to discuss issues and questions with you. Other clinical supervisors assign specific conference times. It is the responsibility of the clinical supervisor to provide a forum for appropriate and effective communication between supervisor and student clinician. However, you share in this responsibility. You may be intimidated by your first clinical supervisor. To complicate matters, because of other obligations, the clinical supervisor may not always be readily available to you. Therefore, it is important to remember that, (1) your supervisor is available for questions, (2) your supervisor is not a mind reader, and (3) that there may be times when you need to be assertive in seeking advice.

Provide Guidelines of Practicum Requirements. Initially, your clinical supervisor will discuss the organization of your clinical practicum with you. He or she will outline expectations of your performance and requirements of your practicum assignment. For example, your supervisor will explain how and when you will be evaluated and on what basis. In addition to requirements of clinical performance, your supervisor will discuss scheduling, attendance, submission of written reports, and mandatory clinical meetings.

Your supervisor should encourage you to discuss any questions or concerns you may have at the beginning of your clinical assignment or as your practicum progresses. As you continue your practicum, issues related to future practicum assignments or requirements may arise. If your clinical supervisor is unavailable or unable to answer your questions (possibly because the supervisor is a part-time member of the university staff), your clinic director or advisor should be able to assist you.

Provide Continuous Feedback. Your clinical supervisor will provide continuous feedback on your clinical performance. Of course, different supervisors have different supervisory styles. One supervisor may give written feedback at the end of each session. Another supervisor may provide verbal feedback or modeling during a session and written feedback after the session. A different supervisor might never interrupt a session unless the well-being of the client is jeopardized. At the beginning of your practicum assignment, your supervisor will discuss the type of feedback he or she will provide.

To maximize learning, client staffings, role playing, or clinical teaching sessions also may be utilized. These sessions may be held on a regular or intermittent basis, before, during, or after clinical practicum sessions.

Informative feedback may take the form of identifying a behavior that the clinician needs to change. For example, beginning clinicians tend to use questions instead of statements—"Can you say /r/?" versus "Say /r/." To give objective feedback, the inappropriate use of questions may be charted by the supervisor.

If you feel that you are not receiving sufficient feedback or that the feedback is unclear, discuss this with your clinical supervisor. Remember, feedback does not necessarily imply negative criticism.

Assist in Planning Clinical Objectives. Typically, your supervisor will direct you to review your clients' charts or case histories and develop an assessment or treatment plan for your first session with your clients. Before your initial meeting with your clients, your supervisor will review these plans with you. The less clinical experience you have had, the more assistance your clinical supervisor will expect you to need.

Your supervisor will help you learn to critically evaluate your clients' speech and language behaviors and learn to develop measurable clinical objectives. Your supervisor also will help you establish priorities for treatment objectives. Chapter 6 describes some general guidelines of selecting target behaviors. Note, however, that your clinical supervisor must approve all major clinical decisions including what to teach and how.

Your supervisor also may identify, or help you identify, personal objectives for you to achieve. You may be asked to describe areas of professional growth and how you plan to achieve it. For example, your supervisor may suggest that you need more information related to the nonverbal child, or you may identify your own weakness in that area when assigned such a child as a client. To supplement your knowledge in this area, your supervisor might direct you to specific resources, or advise you to research the subject area and report your findings to him or her.

Assist in Developing Diagnostic Skills and Assessment Strategies. Your clinical supervisor will observe a minimum of 50% of each evaluation session. You will get feedback on your selection, administration, and interpretation of tests. If necessary, your supervisor may model both general and specific test administration procedures. Your supervisor also will advise you regarding informal observation procedures, client-specific assessment procedures, and assist you in integrating results of standardized test and nonstandardized observations.

Demonstrate a Variety of Clinical Skills. Beginning student clinicians sometimes are unsure of how to implement the myriad of treatment techniques and principles they have observed and read about. For example, if you are exhibiting difficulty with effectively reinforcing a desired behavior, your supervisor will demonstrate the appropriate strategy. Some clinical supervisors prefer to demonstrate with the specific client during treatment sessions. Other supervisors do not interrupt sessions, but may demonstrate a technique after a session and expect you to implement it the following session. Often, supervisors will inform you in advance if they intend to demonstrate a specific technique during a clinical session. You should request demonstration of certain procedures when you do not clearly understand your supervisor's instructions.

Facilitate Development of Client Management Skills. After you develop your treatment goals, you must determine a progression of treatment. Your supervisor will assist you in evaluating the needs of your client including such variables as determining the initial level of treatment, developing intervention strategies, establishing the performance criteria for each level, and accurately charting treatment results. Your supervisor will encourage you to evaluate the effectiveness of each of your clinic sessions and determine what, if any, changes should be made in your treatment goals or strategies.

In evaluating each of your sessions, it is necessary for you and your supervisor to have accurate information on your clients' performance. You will discover that a certain method of charting responses is not appropriate across all clients and that you may need to experiment with different methods. Your supervisor will suggest different ways to maintain accurate records.

In addition to analyzing client performance, you can expect your supervisor to require you to analyze your own behaviors and how they affect client responses. One way your supervisor may assist you in evaluating your performance is by videotaping clinical sessions. You may be required to watch the video independently or jointly with your supervisor. Your supervisor also may chart some of your clinical behaviors (such as your use of positive feedback or method of evoking responses) to show you what you do.

Describe Record Keeping Requirements. As you know, accountability and documentation are important components of clinical service delivery. Certain record-keeping requirements are common across settings and other requirements may be unique to individual sites. Your supervisor will describe the documentation and record-keeping requirements specific to your setting. The methods utilized to ensure confidentiality of clinical records also will be outlined and monitored by your clinical supervisor.

Encourage Independent Problem Solving and Self-Analysis. The importance of the clinical supervisor in providing direct guidance and assistance to student clinicians should not be minimized. Nonetheless, an important role of clinical supervisors is to teach clinicians independent problem-solving skills and self-analysis. Regardless of the number of practicum hours completed, you still will encounter clients exhibiting communicative disorders with which you have had little or no experience. However, if you have developed the ability to critically analyze both your clients' behaviors as well as your own clinical behaviors, you will be able to make appropriate clinical decisions. This is not to suggest that each clinician is, or even should be, highly qualified to work with every type of speech and language disorder. There are clinicians with certain areas of specialization who can better serve specific clients. However, the clinical decision-making process includes knowing when it is necessary to seek additional information or to refer clients to other speech-language pathologists or different professionals.

Your supervisor will provide guidance based on your level of clinical experience. At each level of your practicum experience, your supervisor will involve you in the problem solving and analysis process. The supervisor will make suggestions, but will expect you to expand on those suggestions and to generalize ideas across clients and settings. Your supervisor also will expect you to seek information, rather than just waiting to receive instruction or direction. As you progress in your practicum, your supervisor, while still monitoring your performance, will provide less and less assistance with decision making and allow you to perform with increasing independence.

Help Develop Verbal and Written Skills. Your supervisor will facilitate the development of your verbal and written reporting skills by providing you with opportunities for practicing both types of activities. Content requirements and formats of clinical reports vary across supervisors and settings; therefore, your supervisor should provide you with an outline of the specific professional writing requirements of your assignment.

Although reporting styles may vary, the need to be able to write clear, concise, and logical reports does not. Your supervisor will edit or request that you change reports. Do not be surprised if you must revise a report more than once. When your supervisor first edits your report, the most obvious problems may be noted. However, after these errors are corrected, more subtle problems may be observed requiring you to revise your reports further.

Your supervisor may require you to practice your verbal reporting skills during client staffings, consultation with other professionals, and sharing information with clients and their families. If you have little previous experience with verbal reporting, you might find it beneficial to write out the information you want to cover, and practice presenting it orally. It is also helpful to try to anticipate questions that might arise and prepare answers in advance.

Provide Current Resources. Information is changing rapidly in the field of communicative disorders. Experts continue to suggest new assessment and treatment methods. New instruments and technological devices also are developed frequently . Your supervisor will expect you to use current information, instruments, procedures, and technology and will assist you in locating them. The supervisor will help you research current information and use many campus resources including the library, computer laboratories, writing clinics, and so forth.

Model and Demand Professional Behavior. Your supervisor is a professional and will expect to be treated as one. Your supervisor also will treat you as a professional and expect you to act as one. Also, your supervisor will expect you to know and comply with ASHA's Code of Ethics. Your supervisor will outline the requirements of your clinical site including the dress code, health regulations, and clinical practicum schedule.

Evaluate Your Clinical Work. Your clinical supervisor also is an instructor who must evaluate your clinical work. Every supervisor must strive to make objective and constructive evaluation of your clinical work. Although there may be times set aside for formal evaluations, every time you receive feedback from your supervisor, you will have received some level of evaluation as well.

Help, Guide, and Support You. You can expect your supervisor to be there to help you, guide you, and support you. The supervisor will expect you to have confidence and trust in him or her. Your supervisor is not only your mentor, but also your advocate.

The Off-Campus Clinical Supervisor

Off-campus clinical supervisors may or may not be fully familiar with your university's training program. Consequently, they may not act or hold the same expectations as the supervisors at the university clinic. So, what can you expect and not expect from your off-campus supervisor?

1. **Do expect your off-campus supervisor to perform many of the same activities identified in the previous section:** (1) develop and maintain effective communication; (2) provide guidelines of the practicum requirements; (3) provide on-going feedback; (4) assist in planning clinical goals; (5) assist in developing diagnostic skills; (6) demonstrate

clinical methods; (7) assist in developing client management skills; (8) describe record keeping requirements; (9) encourage independent problem solving; (10) facilitate development of reporting skills; (11) provide current resources; (12) model and demand professional behavior; (13) evaluate your clinical work, and (14) help you and support you. However, you should not expect off-campus clinical supervisors to be exactly the same as the university clinical supervisor in performing all these and other duties.

2. **Do not expect the same frequency of supervision.** The amount of supervision offered at off-campus sites may be more or less. Minimally, the off-campus supervisors will meet ASHA's guidelines for the type and frequency of supervision. However, when you are assigned to an off-campus site, you are expected to be able to work relatively independently, but you may be supervised more closely than when you were less experienced. This increased amount of supervision does not mean that the supervisor does not have much confidence in you. The off-campus supervisors may have only a single student clinician to supervise; whereas, university clinic supervisors may supervise up to four clinicians at one time. The off-campus site also may have additional supervisory requirements to comply with insurance requirements.

3. **Do expect your off-campus supervisor to let you know about the unique aspects of clinical work in his or her setting.** In the beginning, your off-campus supervisor may have to spend extra time in getting you familiarized with the special clinical populations served at the site and the unique clinical and administrative procedures to be followed.

4. **Do expect your supervisor to demand fairly independent performance from you.** This sounds like a contradiction, based on the probability that you will receive greater one-to-one supervision than at the university clinic; however, it is not. Inherent in an internship placement is the assumption that you are fairly advanced and able to make indepen-dent judgments. Because of this, your clinical supervisor certainly will expect you to act relatively independently in planning assessment and treatment sessions, problem solving, researching additional information, and asking necessary questions.

5. **Do not expect your supervisor to know your specific academic background in detail.** Your supervisors at the university clinic probably knew the curriculum content and

orientation of courses you have had. They also knew the level of your clinical experience. But the off-campus supervisors may not be familiar with the full details of the university's training program. They may know what courses you have had, but may not know the scope and orientation of those courses. The supervisors' expectations of you may be based on their general experiences with students of your background. Some supervisors may base expectations on their own educational experiences and the requirements they faced. This is not necessarily a disadvantage, but something of which you should be aware.

Responsibilities of Student Clinicians

Student clinicians must fulfill numerous responsibilities to ensure a successful practicum experience for themselves and to provide effective services to their clients. In essence, though, student clinicians should (a) learn to assess, treat, counsel, and professionally work with their clients and their families; and (b) show systematic progress in their learning of those professional skills.

Throughout the clinical practicum, many of these responsibilities remain unchanged as students progress in their practicum experiences. However, the expectations of the clinical supervisor change. More advanced student clinicians will be expected to fulfill their clinical responsibilities with less guidance from their clinical supervisor. Although individual university departments may have additional requirements, the following sections provide a general overview of the student clinician's responsibilities.

Comply With ASHA's Code of Ethics. In all clinical practicum settings, abide by ASHA's Code of Ethics. It is your responsibility to be aware of the intent of the Code of Ethics and the various principles and proscriptions. The Code of Ethics was discussed in more detail in chapter 3.

Follow Clinic Policies and Procedures. The many clinic policies and procedures student clinicians must follow may appear unwarranted to the new clinician. Yet, these policies and procedures enable the clinic to operate effectively and efficiently. Each clinical site will have different policies and procedures you must follow. Typically, the clinic secretary or your clinical supervisor will let you know the policies. Many practicum sites will have procedural handbooks available to you.

The following subjects commonly are addressed at the university clinic and any off-campus practicum sites: enrolling in clinical practicum, scheduling clients, ensuring client confidentiality, reserving and checking out materials and equipment, maintaining and working with clients' folders, utilizing the clinic telephone, maintaining clinic records, fulfilling insurance and health requirements, and complying with the clinic dress code. If you are unsure of a specific procedure or policy at your clinical site, you must get the information from your clinical supervisor.

Ensure Client Confidentiality. Because of its importance, the necessity of ensuring the client's confidentiality has been addressed in several places in this book. Remember that all information regarding the client is confidential. Do not discuss the client or the client's family by name in public areas. Public areas include reception areas, work rooms, waiting rooms, and other places outside the clinic. Do not leave clients' records unattended at desks or in workrooms. As a general rule, never remove permanent records from the clinic area. Follow the established procedures regarding release of client information to other agencies.

Prepare for Each Clinical Session. Know the administration and evaluation of <u>diagnostic assessment procedures.</u> Review them before every diagnostic session. Inspect the tests you plan to administer before meeting with your client to make sure the tests are complete, that they contain all required materials, and that the necessary test response forms are available. Although it may be another person's job to supply the treatment rooms, it is your responsibility to have all the necessary materials. In the middle of an oral-peripheral examination, you cannot blame someone for not providing the needed supplies. To avoid wasting assessment or treatment time, prepare and organize all materials and forms in advance of each session .

Check in advance any <u>equipment</u> that you plan to use in your clinical sessions to ensure it is working properly. Make sure you know how to operate equipment you plan to use. Some distressing problems can occur with common tape recorders. They may be broken or the batteries may be dead. Not infrequently, student clinicians have recorded an entire clinical session only to find that the pause button was depressed instead of the record button.

Carefully review data obtained in previous sessions to determine appropriate beginning levels and possible sequences of treatment for the sessions for which you are preparing. Make sure the materials you have selected are the most appropriate for the target behaviors you plan to teach. The best organized and most creative materials are ineffective if the target behaviors are inappropriate or unrealistic.

Use Appropriate Diagnostic Instruments. Select and use evaluation procedures and instruments that are appropriate to the client. Select procedures and instruments that are valid, reliable, nonbiased, and comprehensive. The evaluation procedures must sample behaviors adequately. Report with caution the results of tests administered to clients not within the standardization population. Use informal or naturalistic observation of the clients' communicative skills as a part of each evaluation. This type of assessment is used to provide a more comprehensive analysis of the clients' spontaneous speech, and to provide a basis for evaluation when standardized instruments are not appropriate. Standardized tests can supplement information obtained from analysis of the clients' conversational speech.

Develop Measurable Treatment Objectives. Develop measurable treatment objectives based on diagnostic results or reassessment of the client's current communicative skills. You may continue to work on objectives established the previous semester if they still are appropriate for the client. Do not believe erroneously that you are required to develop "original" objectives, even though the previous semester's objectives still are applicable.

Submit Written Assignments Promptly. Your clinical supervisor will notify you of timelines and due dates for written assignments. Each practicum site will have different writing requirements. Writing requirements at the university clinic typically require an initial written summary, daily lesson plans or a semester treatment plan, and a final summary or progress report. Submit written assignments on time, because it is important for many reasons. First, completing assignments on time suggests that you are dependable, and that your practicum assignment is a high priority for you. Second, your written work reflects your knowledge of your clients, their communicative disorders, and of assessment and treatment procedures you plan to implement. A promptly submitted report will help the supervisor give you timely feedback. Third, your reports may suggest to the supervisor the level of supervision you need to work effectively with your client.

Develop an Appropriately Sequenced Treatment Plan. An effective treatment program may fail if it is not properly sequenced for the individual client. For example, if the initial target behavior is defined as the correct production of a phoneme in sentences, you may never get started at all. Therefore, plan and sequence treatment using the initial and continuous assessment data. Plan realistically for the time available within each session. Design maintenance procedures early in the treatment sequence. Include the family in the treatment process. Use clinical procedures based on replicated research and technology. Finally, include the client as an active participant in the intervention process. Read the second part of this textbook for details on treatment procedures.

Maintain Accurate Clinical Records. Maintain an accurate and comprehensive record of your clients' clinical histories and related information in their permanent files. Maintain clinic files in the order established by the clinical site.

Continuous measurement of target responses throughout the treatment sessions and charting them in the form of line or bar graphs will make it easier to see the client's progress, or lack of it. Such graphic and other quantitative measures enable you to find out quickly if treatment is appropriate or if modifications are needed. Graphs also allow you to provide the client (or parent) with a visual representation of progress. Therefore, record and analyze your clients' responses during all assessment and treatment sessions. Learn efficient and accurate charting skills to record the client responses.

Maintain an accurate and complete chronological log of clinical activity. This log is a necessary part of the documentation and analysis process. A review of a client's file should show the client's progress. Record-keeping requirements are discussed in more detail in chapter 5.

Apply Information Learned in Academic Courses to Practicum Assignments. In planning for evaluation and treatment sessions, draw from the information you learned in your academic courses. This seems like a fundamental assumption which should go without mentioning, but occasionally there are students who differentiate between material learned in academic courses and material learned in practicum assignments. Some students fail to see the relevance of what they have learned in classroom to clinical work. The more you are able to integrate academic and clinical assignments, the greater is the value of both. You also will find that information learned in one class that focused on a particular disorder can be expanded on and generalized to other communicative disorders. The information you acquire in your academic studies is the foundation on which you build your independent professional skills and clinical experience.

Research Information. Research information needed to fulfill your clinical assignments. Your clinical supervisor may provide you with resources or you may independently research them. Know the library resources, including current and past periodicals, latest books, and computerized information search programs that are available to find research information. If you are unsuccessful at resolving the clinical question independently, request assistance from your clinical supervisor.

Ask Questions. Though expected to work increasingly independently, you must learn to seek assistance when you have questions. You should not go on with your practicum when you are not sure of something. If you are unclear about clinic policies and procedures, if you are not certain about implementing a specific treatment plan, if you are not sure about directions given by your supervisor, or if you just forgot something that was said, ask for clarification.

Your clinical supervisor does not always immediately know when you need help. If you feel you are not getting enough assistance from your supervisor, evaluate your own behavior before assuming that your supervisor "doesn't have time" or "doesn't care." Some clinical supervisors will be very structured in scheduling times for questions, meetings, and staffings. Others will be less structured and expect student clinicians to approach them with questions as they arise.

Self-Evaluate Clinical Sessions. Do not expect your clinical supervisor to evaluate all your sessions. To make independent clinical judgments, learn to self-evaluate your clinical work. This learning is an essential part of clinical practicum. This skill will enable you to successfully modify evaluation and treatment plans, and to continue to use and expand on information that you acquire throughout your professional career.

There is an ever increasing number of assessment instruments in communicative disorders. To further confuse the student, there are many contradictory theories and treatment strategies. If you can objectively evaluate your clinical behaviors and those of your clients, you can establish the most effective treatment for your clients. Also, you will be better able to find out what academic areas or clinical skills you should target for improvement.

You are not expected to know automatically how to evaluate your clinical sessions. Your supervisor is responsible for helping you acquire this skill.

Maintain Regular Attendance. Attend all scheduled clinical sessions promptly. If you are ill or have a personal emergency, notify your clinical supervisor and, if part of your clinic's protocol, your clients. Studying for examinations, leaving for a vacation, or simply being unprepared are not acceptable reasons for canceling a clinical appointment. Begin and end your clinical sessions on time.

Act Professionally. Sometimes it is difficult to be a student on the one hand and a professional on the other. But remember that though you are under training, you are a professional helping people with communicative disorders.

Know how to make others view you as a professional. Do some of your fellow students generate more of an aura of "professionalism" than others? If you look at their behaviors, you probably will find individuals who have spent much time becoming knowledgeable about their clients' communicative disorders. They will have prepared thoroughly and organized their clinical sessions. They also will have given some thought to how they talk and dress.

Student clinicians who present themselves as professionals also treat their clients, supervisor, clinical staff, and other professionals with respect. In turn, the student clinicians get treated as professionals.

Maintain a Log of Clinical Clock Hours. You are responsible for maintaining a log of the clinical clock hours you have earned. Maintain both a daily and a semester log. University speech and hearing clinics have formats for recording clock hours. Carefully follow the format established at your clinic, because you may not get credit for incorrectly recorded clock hours.

Keep in Touch With Your Clinical Supervisor. You will work with many supervisors. Each may have a different supervisory style. Regardless of your practicum site or the supervisor you have, it is important to maintain contact with your supervisor. If you have any questions or concerns about your assignment, contact your supervisor. If you had a great experience in the clinic, let your supervisor know. Do not expect your supervisor to know everything that happens in each of your sessions. Also, do not expect your supervisor to always know when you need help. Work cooperatively with your supervisor and assume some of the responsibility for maintaining effective communication with him or her.

The interaction between the clinical supervisor and student clinician forms the basis for learning in the practicum setting. To ensure optimal training for the student clinician and quality service for the client, the supervisor and the student clinician should fulfill their respective responsibilities.

5
Working With Clients

T he student clinician's major task is to learn professional skills in working with clients who have communicative disorders. These skills include scheduling clients, evaluating their communicative skills, developing and implementing treatment plans, writing a variety of reports, maintaining adequate records, working with families, and coordinating services with other professionals.

Scheduling Clients

Scheduling clients is one of the initial steps in beginning clinical work. Depending on your clinic's policy, either you or the clinic secretary may schedule your clients. Such factors as the clinician's schedule, client availability, client needs, type of service to be provided, and location of service affect the schedule you develop.

University Clinic Schedules. University clinics schedule clinical sessions based on the availability of clinical supervision, convenience of clients, the schedule of student clinicians, and the operating times of the clinic. Because of the number of variables involved, university clinic schedules may change from semester to semester.

Most university clinics usually operate during regular business hours, Monday through Friday, with some evening sessions available for clients who cannot attend during the day. Clients typically are scheduled for two to three sessions per week. Sessions typically last 30 to 60 minutes. Diagnostic sessions may be scheduled for 1 to 2 hours. Clients are scheduled for individual or group treatment sessions.

At the beginning of the semester (or quarter), you will receive your clinical assignment. You will be given your clinic schedule and your supervisor or clinic director will assign you appropriate clients. Beginning clinicians are assigned one or two clients while the more advanced clinicians may work with three to four clients.

At most schools, student clinicians are responsible for telephoning their clients to schedule them. If one of your clients cannot attend at the proposed time, notify your supervisor and the clinic secretary. You will be assigned another client to contact.

The following general guidelines apply to your initial telephone contact with your client.

1. **Introduce yourself, your credentials and the purpose of your call.** For example, "Hello, this is Jennifer Jones, a graduate student clinician at the University Speech and Hearing Clinic. I'm calling to schedule speech services for your daughter, Lisa." If the client has not been seen previously at your clinic, be prepared to answer questions about the clinic's policies and procedures. New clients will have questions about fees, clinic schedules, parking, the type of supervision provided, the frequency of supervision, qualifications of the supervisors, length of the semester, qualifications of the student clinicians providing services, and related services available (e.g., audiology).

2. **Discuss the client's schedule.** Tell the client when his or her appointment is. Some clinics also may send written appointment cards to clients. If you contact your clients more than five or six days in advance, telephone them again the day before their first appointments to remind them of the date and time. This will help reduce the number of missed appointments.

3. **Clarify ambiguous information and request additional information.** For instance, parents sometimes complete a line incorrectly on the case history; they may write the current date on the line requesting their child's date of birth. Also, request clients or parents to bring all reports from other speech-language pathologists or related specialists they have seen.

4. **Give information about parking permits and clinic fees.** Tell clients where they can park. If a free parking permit is available, tell them how they should get it. If clients state they are unable to afford the clinic fee, ask them to see your clinic director (or, follow the policy already established at your clinic). You do not have the authority to make decisions regarding fee reduction or to set up a payment schedule.

5. **Give directions to the clinic.** New clients may not know where the university clinic is. You are familiar with the campus and may not think in terms of how to get to the clinic from other areas of the community. Therefore, have a map of the campus or city available when you first contact your clients. With the help of the map, give accurate directions. Redundant information is usually helpful to the individual unfamiliar with the campus. For example, you might say, "then turn left on Lakeview, you'll be going east. Go to the third stoplight which is Trout Avenue, and turn right, then you'll be heading north."

6. **Give directions to the clinic waiting room.** Tell your clients that you will meet them in the waiting room after they have completed their business at the clinic office. Each clinic has its procedures for the first meeting with clients. Follow the procedures at your university.

7. **Ensure the client has the correct appointment date and time before ending the phone call.** After you have answered the clients' questions and given directions, tell them you will see them at the appointed date, time, and place. "O.K., I'll see you on Monday, September 2nd at 9:00 a.m. at the clinic waiting room."

Hospital Schedules. In medical settings, inpatients often are scheduled for speech services 5 days a week, Monday through Friday. Attempts are made to schedule services at times that are most beneficial to patients. Patients may be seen one or two times a day. Their schedules are dependent on the length of time they are able to effectively participate in evaluation or treatment. For example, clients may have been prescribed speech-language services five times per week for an hour each day. But, if they are unable to attend for a full hour, they may be seen for 30 minutes during the morning and again for 30 minutes during the afternoon.

Other variables also must be considered. Though your hospital assignment may require you to begin at 8:00 a.m., you actually may not begin direct patient contact until 9:00 or 9:30 a.m. Much of the patient care occurs early in the morning. This care may include such activities as administering medications, providing breakfast, toileting, and bathing. Therefore, you must coordinate your schedule with the nursing staff.

Coordination with other patient rehabilitation services also is necessary. For example, besides speech services, a patient may be receiving physical and occupational therapies.

Also, it may be necessary to adjust the patient's schedule around a regular family visiting time. Though you want to involve the family in your patient's treatment, there should be times when the family can be with the patient to just visit. There is the occasional family member who can be at the hospital only at a certain time because of transportation, work, or school obligations.

After you have consulted with other staff and determined a schedule of therapy for your patient, remain with the same schedule as much as possible. As patients are discharged and new patients enrolled, some schedule changes will be necessary.

You also must allow time in your daily schedule for indirect services. Schedule time for report writing, consultation with other professionals, family consultation, and your own breaks and lunches.

If you are working in an **outpatient setting**, the receptionist or secretary may schedule your clients. As much as possible, clients are scheduled for a regular time during their entire enrollment. For example, one of your clients may be scheduled for speech services every Monday, Wednesday, and Friday from 10:00 to 10:45 a.m. This schedule may not fluctuate from week to week.

School Schedules. In the educational setting, caseloads sometimes are large and several service delivery models are used. Because of this, scheduling may seem overwhelming to the beginning clinician.

First, you must determine what type of schedule you will implement. The two common types of schedules are block (intensive cycle) and intermittent. In block scheduling, specific students (or schools) receive services 5 days a week for a certain number of weeks (for example, 6 weeks). After the predetermined length of time, service is rotated to the next group of students (or schools). In intermittent scheduling, all students and schools are served each week. For example, the speech-language pathologist assigned to serve two schools might provide services on Mondays and Wednesdays at one school, and Tuesdays, Thursdays, and Fridays at the other school.

Second, your schedule will be influenced by the service delivery model used. Many school clinicians provide a combination of the traditional pull-out model, consultation model, and classroom-collaboration model. Each model requires different amounts of time and considerable coordination with the other professionals involved. These models were discussed in more detail in chapter 2.

Third, you must determine how often each student on your caseload will receive service. You also must determine if they will receive treatment individually or in a group.

Fourth, school and class schedules must be considered. You must find out the times of recess, lunch, class dismissal, school assemblies, and so on. Several of your students may be receiving services from other professionals including the school psychologist, resource specialist, adaptive physical education specialist, or physical therapist. There also will be certain periods of the class that the teacher does not want the student to miss on a regular basis.

Appropriate implementation of any type of schedule requires effective communication with the classroom teacher and other specialists serving the student on your caseload. When you participate in your school internship, your supervisory clinician or the university supervisor will provide you with practice in scheduling and decision making regarding scheduling options.

Summary of Scheduling Guidelines. Because of the number of factors involved, scheduling a client (or patient, or student) can become an art form of its own. Although frequency of service and procedures for scheduling clients will differ across settings, the following are common factors to include in implementing your schedule at any practicum site.

1. Schedule sessions to optimize the effectiveness of treatment. Make decisions about time of day, length of session, frequency of treatment, group or individual treatment, and direct or indirect (e.g., consultative) service delivery. In making your decisions, follow the clinic guidelines on these matters.
2. Coordinate speech-language pathology service with other individuals providing services for your client.
3. Follow your schedule. Be punctual in beginning and ending sessions. Alter your schedule as little as possible, and communicate any changes in your schedule to all individuals affected by the change.
4. Allow time in your schedule for paperwork, evaluations, conferences, and breaks.

Assessment of Clients

Prior to being enrolled for treatment of communicative disorders, individuals must have a complete speech-language assessment. The assessment allows you to determine if a communicative disorder exists, and, if it does, the nature and extent of that disorder. In addition, the evaluation allows you to gather enough information to include recommendations on possible treatment objectives, treatment procedures, and timelines for treatment.

Many university training programs have a "diagnostic clinic" designed for the sole purpose of evaluation. Other clinical settings may have clinicians who perform only assessments and are not involved in treatment. However, most speech-language pathologists are involved in both assessment and treatment.

It is not the purpose of this section to provide a comprehensive assessment guide, but to give an overview of the components of evaluation with emphasis on the university clinic setting. Read one of the many excellent books on evaluation and diagnosis (Darley & Spriestersbach, 1978; Emerick & Haynes, 1986; Peterson & Marquardt, 1990).

Assessments at the University Clinic. At the university clinic, the initial assessment procedure begins after an individual has contacted the clinic regarding a communication problem. Assessment procedures vary depending on disorders, clients, and clinicians. However, the following procedures are common to all assessments.

1. **Obtain a case history.** A completed case history form is required prior to scheduling an individual for an evaluation. Occasionally, the clinician and client may complete the case history during the initial interview. The case history can be very extensive and often includes: prenatal, birth, and developmental information; medical, social, educational, and occupational history; and, previous related evaluation and treatment results. Following receipt of the necessary information in the clinic office, an evaluation is scheduled.

2. **Interview the client (or parent).** The interview allows you to clarify information reported on the case history and obtain additional information either omitted or inferred from the case history. Information obtained during the interview also suggests the types of testing that you will need to perform. Also, the interview is an information-giving process in which

you explain the assessment procedures and results to the client, parents, or both.

Each interview will vary depending on the type of disorder, related problems, and so on. Some interviews will be relatively short, and others may be lengthy. Typically, the more complicated the medical history, the longer the interview. You also may be involved in a lengthy interview with clients who have received treatment from other agencies. Interviews also may have different formats. To assess the communication skills of a child, you will interview the parent. You may or may not include the child in the interview. You may want to include the child with a fluency disorder in the interview; whereas, a language disordered child may not be able to participate in the interview because of limited expressive vocabulary.

Beginning clinicians sometimes experience two problems in the interview. Both are usually due to the reliance on a preset interview format.

First, it is not uncommon for beginning student clinicians to have some difficulty establishing rapport with their clients during the interview. This is sometimes due to the inappropriate use of closed ended questions and the use of the case history form as an interview guide. Following the case history line by line, beginning clinicians sometimes question the client even though the client has already responded to these questions on the case history. For example, you might ask, "Has Josh had ear infections? Has he had any seizures? Has Josh had mumps?", and so on. Generally, it is more effective to summarize information on the case history and request verification. For example, "You noted on the case history that Josh was sick for several weeks as an infant. Tell me a little bit more about that." This is not to imply that you should not ensure that all necessary information is accurately supplied, but redundant questions should be avoided.

Second, ignoring, or missing, important information is another problem related to relying on an interview "script." For example, you may ask a question about educational history, "What grade is Josh in?" By waiting only for the response to the question in order to pursue the next question, you may miss important information that the parent reports. It is important to direct the interview, but it is equally important to listen and respond to what is said in the interview. Appendix D contains a sample of an interview.

3. **Perform an oral-peripheral examination.** An oral-peripheral examination is performed to investigate the structural and functional integrity of the speech mechanism. You should systematically evaluate the oral-peripheral mechanism during each examination to avoid overlooking any areas. That is, always evaluate structures in a certain sequence. For example, some clinicians begin with general facial features, then progress to examination of the lips, teeth, tongue, hard palate, and so on. Other clinicians begin examining the oral cavity first and then examine peripheral areas.

   It is helpful to orally record the evaluation (i.e., verbally describe your observations while audiotaping). This step will allow you to continue the examination without having to stop and write notes.

   Occasionally, a child will refuse to allow invasive procedures during the oral examination. In this case, you can observe the speech mechanism during activities such as laughing, speaking, and eating. Perform the examination later in the evaluation session or in a treatment session if the child is enrolled for speech services.

4. **Screen the client's hearing.** ASHA guidelines require an audiometric screening as part of a complete speech and language assessment. University clinics routinely screen the hearing of clients as part of a speech and language assessment. In other practicum settings, an audiometer may not be available to the speech-language pathologist. Therefore, the clients are referred to an audiologist. In the public school setting, the school nurse, licensed as an audiometrist, often performs hearing screenings. Before evaluating individuals wearing hearing aids, it is important to find out when they had their last audiological evaluation. Also, perform a hearing aid check to determine if the hearing aid is functioning.

5. **Obtain speech-language samples.** The speech sample is sometimes referred to as an "informal" assessment procedure which seems to diminish the importance of analysis of the sample. However, the conversational speech sample is one of the most important assessment instruments available to you. It allows you to evaluate your client's communicative abilities in a natural context. It is essential to the assessment of a client's actual speech and language performance. To ensure the reliability of the speech sample, you should obtain more than one sample. Direct conversation to provide clients opportunities to produce a variety of language structures

(e.g., declaratives, interrogatives, different verb tenses, and so forth.) If possible, sample conversation in a variety of environments. In adult evaluations, the interview commonly is used to obtain at least a portion of the conversational sample. At the university clinic, other environments can be sampled easily. Sample clients' speech while they are speaking on the telephone, speaking with the clinic receptionist, or speaking with a bookstore salesperson.

Include more than just the client's mean length of utterance in your analysis of the speech sample. Include information about the client's semantic, morphologic, syntactic, and pragmatic productions. In addition to analysis of language, you will use the speech samples to examine articulation skills. Compute overall speech intelligibility. Analyze production of phonemes. Note specific errored phonemes, types of errors (e.g., omissions, substitutions, distortions), frequency of errors, and percentage of occurrence. You also may describe specific error patterns (e.g., syllable reduction, cluster reduction, fronting). Observe voice characteristics: quality, pitch, intensity. Note such behaviors as the number of pitch breaks in a 5-minute speech sample, or the absence of adequate breath support. Measure the types and frequency of dysfluencies in the sample and calculate the dysfluency rate. Refer to Appendix E for discussion on types of dysfluencies and how to calculate them.

To evoke conversation, clinicians evaluating children often use pictures, books, and toys. The recurring problem with pictures is that they often evoke single word responses. Using books typically does not result in an adequate conversation sample. Children often prefer to look at the pictures rather than talk to the clinician. You can use toys to gather a speech sample; however, again, some children become involved in playing with the toys and do not engage in conversation. Before bringing out pictures and books for children to describe, try to involve them in conversation. If a child is school age, ask about most and least favorite school activities, favorite teachers, what happens to students who get in trouble in the cafeteria, best friends, school bully, and so on. The preschool child may respond to similar questions about preschool or siblings, educational programs on television, cartoon shows, and so forth. Sometimes, you can tell the child something about yourself first to stimulate speech. For example, "I have a puppy that is so silly. Yesterday he ran through the sprinklers and then came and jumped all over me! Tell me about your puppy."

If possible, audiotape or videotape a short conversational sample between a parent and child while they are in the room alone. Tell parents why and what you are doing. Ask them to talk (or play) with their children as they would normally.

Ask parents to maintain a daily log of their children's speech for one week. This is one way to get a more complete view of the language of a young child who is reluctant to participate in activities in the clinic. Though the information may not be fully accurate, it will give you a better idea of the child's language performance as well as an idea of the parent's perception of the child's communication skills. A parent may report that his or her child uses only single words. However, while recording the child's speech for a week, the parent may find that the child is using some two-word phrases. Another parent might report that his or her child has a large vocabulary. The record of verbal productions may confirm or contradict this report. Refer to Appendix F for information on obtaining and analyzing speech samples.

6. **Administer standardized tests.** There are a number of standardized tests designed to evaluate communicative disorders. Standardized tests can be used to substantiate your clinical observations, but should not be used to replace those observations. Test selection must be appropriate for the client. Tests must be reliable, valid, and culturally nonbiased. They should adequately sample behaviors. Review tests before administering them. You must know the administration and scoring procedures. If you have to concentrate on remembering administration or scoring procedures to the exclusion of observing your client, you may miss important behaviors exhibited by the client. For example, if you are unfamiliar with the Peabody Picture Vocabulary Test, you may be busy figuring out basals and ceilings and miss the child's perseverative responses or uncooperative behaviors. It is important to remember that the information obtained from a standardized test is only as good as the examiner.

7. **Use other evaluation instruments.** Technology is providing speech-language pathologists with an increasing number of computerized equipment to quantify data that were previously evaluated subjectively. If equipment such as the Visi-Pitch, Nasometer, or Computerized Speech Lab are

available at your university clinic or practicum setting, take the time to learn and use them.

Depending on the type of disorder you evaluate, other types of testing and sampling may be performed. For example, you will assess stimulability of misarticulated sounds in evaluation of articulation disorders. You may analyze reading samples in your assessments of fluency disorders.

8. **Discuss impressions and recommendations.** After you have obtained all the necessary data on your client's communicative abilities, analyze and summarize the assessment results. Find out what all the test scores, the oral-peripheral exam, and speech sample results mean. It is not sufficient to report only test scores without also making both objective and subjective clinical observations. These observations are discussed with the client at the end of the assessment. You may report the observations in the body of your written report, or summarize them at the end of your report. Based on your analysis of the client's speech and language skills, make recommendations for or against treatment. If treatment is recommended, report to the client specific objectives, prognosis for obtaining the objectives, and possible duration of treatment. If treatment is not recommended, state clearly the rationale for not recommending treatment. Discuss your assessment plans with your clinical supervisor before meeting with your clients. Also, notify your supervisor of the time of the scheduled evaluation. As you know, ASHA mandates that 50% of each diagnostic session be supervised by your supervisor.

Reassessment of Clients

Treatment efficacy and client progress are continuously assessed through accurate record keeping, probes, and self-evaluations. Specific tests may be administered at the clinician's (or supervisor's) discretion.

Clients returning to the university clinic for another term of treatment should be reassessed before continuing treatment. A reassessment of all areas of speech and language typically is unnecessary. For example, it is not necessary to readminister a battery of language tests to a client diagnosed with a fluency disorder who had no previous indications of a language problem. Important reassessment data needed for the continuing client may be the results of a speech sample, hearing screening, oral examination, course of the disorder in the absence of treatment, and baselines of target behaviors. See chapter 7 for procedures for establishing baselines.

Additional procedures and timelines for assessment and reassessment of clients are mandated by insurance companies and the public schools. Find out from your supervisor about these procedures and timelines.

Establishing a Working Relationship With the Client and the Family

To treat clients effectively, you should establish a good working relationship with the client and the family. Individuals with communicative disorders and their families initially may feel uncomfortable with the treatment process. They may not know much about the treatment, its duration, and its effects. Clients and their families may not begin treatment with the same level of knowledge or enthusiasm that student clinicians do. Therefore, you should educate clients and their families about their responsibilities, the treatment procedures, and their effects. To this end, you must establish good communication between yourself, your client, and your client's family. Because you are learning to do this, you also should maintain constant communication with your clinical supervisor.

Before you discuss important issues with your clients, obtain your supervisor's approval. When you do not know the answer to your clients' or their families' questions, tell them that you will find out from your supervisor. Then, discuss the questions with your supervisor and find out how to answer them. On occasions, because of the complexity of the information to be presented, your supervisor may decide that he or she needs to talk with the family. In such cases, the supervisor will probably include you in the discussion so you will learn to handle such issues.

At the beginning, give clients or families an overview of assessment or reassessment results, the planned treatment, expected results, what the family members should do at home, and follow-up and booster treatment procedures. In talking with clients and their parents, use simple, direct language. Do not give obscure answers that are couched in incomprehensible jargon. When you need to use technical terms, describe them, define them, and give everyday examples. However, do not talk down to people. For example, when the father of a child who is language delayed is a professor of English, do not try to explain prepositions that you want to teach the child. Similarly, if the mother of a child is a physician, do not try to describe the velopharyngeal mechanism in everyday language.

Always give accurate information. Do not bluff. An often asked question is what caused the speech or language problem? Why does my son stutter? Why can't my youngest child talk, while two older children are doing fine? The parents assume that research will have provided answers. But the research information may not provide a clear-cut answer that satisfies clients or their family.

You can tell parents and clients that it is difficult to point out the cause of a disorder in a given client. Our knowledge of disorders and their potential causes are applied to groups of persons, not to specific individuals. For example, you can say that we know many potential causes of stuttering including hereditary predisposition, faulty learning, environmental stress, instability in the nervous system, and many others. But clinicians cannot say why a given child or adult stutters, because several factors may come together to produce a problem.

Discuss the sequence of treatment with your clients. Explain that treatment will begin at a simpler level and progress gradually to more complex levels. For example, "I will begin training the /s/ sound in single words. First, I will teach the sound at the beginning of words. After Jason masters the sound in words, he will learn to use them in phrases and sentences. Finally, Jason will learn to produce the sounds correctly in conversation—here at the clinic and at home and school." Explain too that, although a target behavior may be established quickly in the clinical setting, it takes additional work to establish that behavior in everyday communicative situations. Allow the client, the family members, or both sufficient time to express concerns or ask questions.

Answer questions about the treatment outcome in probabilistic terms. You may tell the parents that they may see some improvements in their child's fluency after 3 months of treatment, but you may not say that "John will be speaking fluently in 6 months." Point out to parents that the effect of treatment will depend on many factors including the motivation of the client, the amount of family support, duration of treatment, and so forth. Recall that ASHA Code of Ethics asks you not to guarantee treatment outcome.

Ask family members to observe treatment sessions. This helps the family to understand the treatment process and the abilities of the client. Allow them time to discuss what they see with you. Answer questions that the family may have and give information to begin integrating the family into the therapeutic process. Be sure to tell the client and family that their questions and input are always welcome.

Regularly review your clients' progress with their families. Give periodic progress reports to parents of child clients. Discuss their child's progress only in the treatment room. Avoid discussions in the hallway, waiting room, and such other places because they compromise client confidentiality. Also, such discussions usually are hurried and noncommunicative.

The ultimate goal of treatment is to integrate the behaviors trained in the clinical setting into the client's everyday communicative environment. To do this, it is necessary for you to work closely with the client's family so that they support the newly established communicative behaviors at home and in other nonclinical settings. Maintenance strategies are described in chapter 9.

Report Writing

There are many different types of written reports used in the evaluation and treatment of communicative disorders. Diagnostic reports provide comprehensive information on a client's pretreatment status. Treatment plans describe short- and long-term goals and the procedures used to obtain those goals. Lesson plans describe treatment planned for one or a few sessions. Client performance is described in different formats, including progress reports, final summaries, and discharge reports.

In addition to generic reports, public agencies have specific reporting requirements. Individualized Education Programs (IEPs) are required in the public schools for individuals with disabilities, 3 through 21 years of age. The Individual Family Service Plan (IFSP) is required for individuals with disabilities, birth through 2 years of age and their families.

The general format and content of a variety of reports are discussed in the following sections. At each practicum site, you should find out what specific reporting procedures must be followed.

General Guidelines on Report Writing

Written reports document the status of a client and thus provide a basis for future comparisons. Also, they provide an efficient form of communication with other individuals. In clinical training programs, supervisors judge a student's knowledge and writing skills by his or her written reports. Besides, many different individuals including allied health professionals, educators, clients, and the clients' family members also read the reports. Each person who reads a clinical report is likely to make certain assumptions regarding the clinician's training and professional skills.

Although content is the most important element of your report, clear, concise presentation, neatness, and accurate use of vocabulary, grammar, spelling, and punctuation also are important. In fact, probably the first impression formed of your report is based on how the report looks, which may or may not have anything to do with your clinical abilities. As a general rule, consider the following in writing reports.

1. Write in complete sentences.
2. Spell all words correctly.
3. Use correct punctuation.
4. Present information in a logical sequence.
5. Do not use nebulous or ambiguous statements.
6. Provide as much detail necessary to clearly describe the client's communicative abilities.
7. Avoid making inferential judgments without substantiating data or qualifying statements.
8. Avoid the use of jargon.
9. Avoid the use of such qualifiers as *like, very, rather*, and so on.
10. Do not use sexist or culturally biased statements.
11. Use correct margins and line spacing. Follow the format requested by your supervisor.
12. Use the required type of paper. Most clinics require you to use nonerasable white bond paper. However, initial drafts of reports may be typed or printed on lower grade paper.
13. Typewritten pages and computer printouts should be easy to read. Print should be dark. Discard (or recycle) ribbons and cartridges that are worn out.
14. Proofread your reports before submitting them.

Some beginning student clinicians may not know where or how to begin their first reports. The university clinic often requires more detailed reports than are typically required (or necessary) at other practicum sites. The rationale behind the overly detailed reports is that if information is not included in the report, then possibly, you did not observe or consider it. Also, if you know how to write a detailed report well, you can always write brief reports equally well.

The following sections offer guidelines for you to write different kinds of reports. Follow the requirements on the format, style, and content of reports specified at each of your practicum sites.

Treatment Plans

After the assessment is completed, write treatment plans that describe short- and long-term objectives and the procedures for achieving those objectives. A well-written treatment plan and accurate progress notes will allow another clinician to review the client's records and begin treatment based on the supplied information. ASHA's Professional Services Board (1984) requires written treatment plans that are reviewed and changed as the client's needs change. ASHA recommends that the discussion of the treatment plan with the client and the client's family be noted on the treatment record. ASHA states that the following information should be contained in a treatment plan.

1. Prognostic statements.
2. Written long- and short-term objectives based on conclusions and recommendations of an evaluation.
3. Statements regarding type, frequency, and duration of treatment.

In addition to this information, treatment plans include descriptions of target behaviors, stimuli to evoke responses, topographical aspects of responses, performance criteria, response consequences, probes, generalization and maintenance training, dismissal criteria, and follow-up treatment. This information is detailed in the following section.

The preparation and writing of treatment plans will vary from setting to setting. Public schools, clinics, and insurance companies have their own formats. In the following section, common components of treatment plans will be presented along with examples specific to certain clinical settings. You are likely to receive additional instructions at individual practicum sites.

Writing a Treatment Plan. The comprehensive treatment plan describes treatment from the beginning of treatment to maintenance of trained behaviors in natural environments. It details both the client's performance and the clinician's performance, as well as the interaction between the two (Hegde, 1985).

The treatment plan does not have to be lengthy, but it should be comprehensive. When you write a treatment plan, do the following (Hegde, 1985).

1. **Briefly summarize identification data.** Describe background information, current performance levels, and purpose of treatment.
2. **Describe target behaviors.** Include both long- and short-term objectives in your description. You must write objectives that are client specific (that is, appropriate and useful to the client), valid, measurable behaviors. Chapter 6 provides information on the selection of target behaviors. Ideally, you will have established baselines of target behaviors before preparing a treatment plan.
3. **Describe stimuli to evoke responses.** You must determine if pictures, objects, conversation, or orthographic symbols will be used to obtain a specific response. You also must decide if visual, auditory, or tactile stimulation will be used. You must identify the setting in which training will be performed (e.g., in the clinical setting, in the client's home, and so on). It is not uncommon for training to begin at a single word level with the presentation of pictures in the clinical setting and advance to the spontaneous speech level with conversational interaction in extraclinical environments.
4. **Describe topographical aspects of responses.** Response topography identifies the level at which training is initiated (e.g., at the syllable level) and the levels of progression. Response topography is not disorder specific, but is used in treatment across all communication disorders. For example, a client with a voice disorder may only be able to sustain an appropriate pitch during single word productions. A client with an articulation disorder may only be able to produce the target phoneme accurately at the single word level.
5. **Specify performance criteria.** Describe the rate of accuracy that will be accepted as the criterion for moving through the training hierarchy. Distinguish between modeled and evoked responses.
6. **Describe response consequences.** Describe how you increase desirable behaviors and decrease undesirable behaviors. Specify any treatment modifications in the progress report or final summary. Response consequences that

increase or decrease behaviors are discussed in chapters 7 and 8, respectively.

7. **Describe probes.** Probes are designed to evaluate generalization of trained behaviors. However, they frequently are absent from treatment plans, perhaps because some clinicians feel they are implied within the training sequence. To ensure that probes are not omitted, describe their use in the treatment plan. Answer the following questions in describing probes: When will probes be administered? What type of probe will be utilized? What is the criterion? What happens if the criterion is or is not met? See chapter 7 for details on probe procedures. Appendix G has a sample probe procedure and recording sheet.

8. **Describe generalization and maintenance.** Describe how you measure generalization (through probes) and how you program maintenance of target behaviors. Include in the description how you plan to train other individuals in the client's environment.

9. **Describe dismissal criterion.** This criterion typically reflects production of the target behaviors in conversational speech in both clinical and extraclinical settings. Written dismissal criterion helps ensure accountability. See chapter 7 for recommended criterion.

10. **Describe follow-up or booster treatment.** After clients have met a certain performance criteria, they are dismissed from frequently scheduled treatment sessions. However, many clients require "booster" or "follow-up" sessions in order to maintain a certain proficiency level. For example, a fluency client who has established 98% fluent speech in clinical and extraclinical settings may be dismissed from twice-a-week treatment sessions. However, he or she should be scheduled for periodic follow-up sessions to assist in maintenance of fluency skills. You should specify the intervals for follow-up sessions in your initial treatment plan. Refer to Appendix H for a sample treatment plan.

Writing Lesson Plans. Though you have written a comprehensive treatment plan, write session-by-session or weekly lesson plans so the supervisor knows what you are doing in a given session. As part of your planning and preparation for clinical sessions, you will write lesson plans for each of your clients. At the university clinic, lesson plans commonly are developed on a weekly basis and submitted to the clinical supervisor in advance for approval. The lesson plan typically contains the following information:

1. **Treatment objectives.** Write the treatment objectives for your client. For example: *The production of /s/ in word initial positions at the evoked level, with 90% accuracy.*
2. **Procedures and materials for obtaining the objectives.** Describe how you will implement the treatment objectives, include materials and treatment procedures. For example: *The /s/ picture cards and /s/ objects will be presented to the client. The client will be required to name each picture. All correct /s/ productions will be verbally reinforced. All incorrect /s/ productions will be interrupted by a verbal "No" or "Stop."*

Information contained in the lesson plan may be similar to items identified in the treatment plan (e.g., response typography, criterion levels, management of consequences). However, the lesson plan does not always allow for a complete view of the client's treatment. The lesson plan describes what is done in a session or two, whereas the treatment plan describes the total sequence of treatment for a given period. Refer to Appendix I for a sample lesson plan.

Writing Individualized Educational Programs. The Public Law 94-142 (and its amendments) mandates a free, appropriate public education and related services for all children and youth who are handicapped. Speech-language pathology is a part of Designated Instructional Services (DIS) under special education services. A written Individualized Educational Program (IEP) is required for each child, ages 3 through 21 years, who receives special education services.

IEP's originally were formulated to provide for management, communication, and accountability in special education services. The IEP is more of a management plan than a treatment plan. The IEP describes what will be trained but not the specific training procedures. Specific rules regulate the development, writing, and implementation of IEPs. There are many legal requirements regarding the timelines for services, identification, referral, assessment, enrollment and dismissal of students, the rights of parents, and due process. The following section gives you guidelines on writing the speech-language IEP.

Content of the IEP. A speech-language pathologist writes an IEP for each student he or she serves. The parents are members of the IEP team and provide input regarding the delivery of special education services for their children. An IEP must be developed before a student can receive services. An annual meeting to review the IEP is required, although meetings may be held more frequently. Many IEP forms are used, but the basic content is the same. To provide a comprehensive management plan, the following information must be included on an IEP (Dublinske, 1978; California State Department of Education, 1989).

1. **Give the identifying information.** List the child's name, address, phone number, birthdate, and parent's name(s) on the IEP. Also, write the student identification or folder number on the IEP. Note the child's grade, primary language, and English language proficiency on the IEP.

2. **Describe the child's present levels of performance.** State current communicative abilities, including both receptive and expressive speech and language skills, behavioral problems noted or reported, related educational strengths or weaknesses, and contributing historical or current developmental or health information. Present levels of performance must be based on at least two assessment procedures. Report test scores as standard scores or percentiles. Both standardized tests and speech samples typically are utilized to describe communicative skills. Sometimes you may refer the reader to a separate diagnostic report rather than repeating the information. (e.g., you might write: *For additional information, see diagnostic report 4-10-91.*) You must report the child's present levels of performance as compared to educational performance. For instance, report how the 6 year old child's speech intelligibility of 50% affects his or her educational performance. Report sufficient information to develop appropriate objectives.

3. **Describe objectives.** List long-term goals to describe the child's expected performance for an entire school year. Objectives (or short-term goals) reflect steps necessary to obtain the long-term goal. Write measurable objectives that have a completion date, and performance criteria. For example: *Goal: Increase sentence length in conversation to a minimum mean length of utterance of 4.0 words by _____(specifiy a date).*
Objective: By _____(specify a date), following picture presentation, Jennie will produce 10 sentences, containing

a minimum of 4 words, with 90% accuracy at the evoked level over three sessions. Progress will be measured by clinician charting.

Base the long-term goals and the objectives on information reported in the present levels of performance. You will guide the selection of appropriate goals and objectives. However, other IEP team members, especially the parents, provide input regarding the development of the student's IEP goals and objectives. At the annual review meeting, note the status of the goals and objectives. Some of these may have been met, others may not have been met. Work on some goals may not have begun yet. There is no required number of goals or objectives.

4. **Describe special education services required.** Specify the type of service that will be provided, the frequency of the service, and the duration of each session on the IEP. For example, speech services may be provided as follows:
   Group therapy/2x's per week/40 minutes each session.
   or
   Teacher consult/1x per month/30 minutes each session.

5. **Describe the amount of time the child will spend in the regular educational program.** Note the child's participation in regular education on the IEP. For the Speech IEP, you may abbreviate the amount of time the child will spend in regular education as a percentage, such as: *95% per week.* You may also list it as an exclusion (i.e., all the time except the time they spend in speech): *all but 2x's per week/ 40 minutes each session.*

6. **Describe when the services will begin and end.** Write the beginning and ending dates of service on the IEP. Services should begin with minimal delay. Initiation of service often begins the next school day, or week, after the IEP meeting. If an IEP meeting is held at the end of the school year, services begin as soon as school resumes. Because an annual review is required of each student enrolled in special education services, you must write the duration of service for 1 year or less. Note this in month/day/year format (e.g., 11/10/92).

7. **Specify the rationale for special education services.** The rationale or justification for service is based on an established criteria for enrollment. In an IEP, indicate if the child is to be enrolled in, continued, or dismissed from special education services.

The criteria for speech-language pathology services are based on legal requirements and are not always consistent with common practices in the community. As noted before, a 5-year-old child with a frontal lisp may receive speech-language pathology services through a private agency, but may not be eligible for speech services in the school until he or she has reached the age of 8. Your school district will provide you with a summary of their eligibility criteria for speech-language pathology services.

The justification for service can be brief or lengthy:

(a) *Language needs cannot be met in the regular education setting. Standardized test scores reflected performance 1.5 standard deviations below the mean in all language areas. Analysis of a conversation sample revealed errors in syntax and morphology and limited semantic abilities.*

(b) *Conversational speech is 15% dysfluent. Speech needs cannot be met in the regular education classroom.*

8. **Describe all professionals providing services.** The child receiving speech-language pathology services also may be receiving other special education services. Give the names of all services and all service providers on the IEP. Following is an example of a list of services and the individuals responsible for providing the service:

- Counseling—School Psychologist
- Medication follow-up—School Nurse
- Speech services—School speech-language pathologist

9. **Get the signature of all individuals attending the IEP meeting.** The names, positions, signatures, and dates of participation of all the individuals attending the IEP meeting must appear on the IEP. Get the parents' signatures on the IEP indicating consent with the IEP for their child's placement in special education. Parents dissenting with the recommended IEP may be provided a separate line to sign or box to check, but a signature may still be required to indicate attendance at the meeting. The child may also attend and be a member of

the IEP team. If appropriate, have the child sign the IEP form. If an interpreter is used at the IEP meeting, get the interpreter's signature and write his or her title on the IEP.

10. **Note additional IEP information.** Write (or check) the following information on the IEP:

  - Date of annual review.
  - Date of 3-year evaluation.
  - Eligibility for extended school year.
  - Recommendations for specific materials, methods, or equipment needed to accomplish the goals.

To reduce paperwork, many school districts use computerized forms or checklists for their IEPs. The computer generated and checklist formats should be diverse enough to allow the development of an "individualized program." This is not a problem with most programs. If none of the prewritten objectives are appropriate, there usually is a space for "other" objectives to be written. Your school site will supply you with IEP forms.

Individual Family Service Plans. As an amendment to PL 94-142, Public Law 99-457 (Part H) established an early intervention program for infants and toddlers and their families. This program requires that an Individual Family Service Plan (IFSP) be written for children with disabilities, ages birth through 2 years. The IFSP must be developed by a multidisciplinary team of professionals and the child's parent(s). The IFSP contains the following information.

1. Present levels of performance (physical, cognitive, communicative, and self-help).
2. Family needs and strengths related to assisting the child.
3. Intervention goals and the way progress will be measured.
4. Types of services the child will receive.
5. Initiation and duration of services.
6. The name of the case manager.

The IEP and IFSP are similar in that they both describe clinical and educational objectives, types of services to be provided, and the beginning and ending dates of services. The IFSP differs from the IEP because of its emphasis on family involvement. The IFSP targets not only the needs of the child, but the strengths and weaknesses of the family and how these influence the child's development. The IFSP incorporates public school services and the services of other public agencies (e.g., families may need respite care services, or social welfare services, as well as educational and rehabilitation services). The case manager is selected based on the needs of the child and the family. The case manager basically is responsible for identifying, coordinating, and monitoring services. The case manager may be a speech-language pathologist, audiologist, special education teacher, psychologist, social worker or other professional. A review of the IFSP is required every 6 months, compared with the IEP's annual review.

Diagnostic Reports

Diagnostic reports are written following the evaluation of a client. A diagnostic report is a summary of case history, assessment data, clinical impressions, conclusions, and recommendations. It provides a clear, written statement of the client's communicative abilities at the time of the evaluation. It also provides a forum for communicating with other professionals. The diagnostic report sometimes is used for research; therefore, it is important to document information clearly and differentiate between subjective statements and objective data.

Each client's file must contain a diagnostic evaluation. A copy of an evaluation performed at another facility may be included in a case file (ASHA Professional Services Board, 1984). When you are assigned a client who has been evaluated by another clinician, obtain a copy of the diagnostic report for the client's file.

There are several formats for writing diagnostic reports (Darley & Spriestersbach, 1978; Emerick & Haynes, 1986; Flower, 1984; Knepflar & May, 1989). In addition, reporting requirements vary at each practicum site. To write a diagnostic report, use the following outline, or modify it for different practicum settings.

1. **Give identification information.** Give this information at the beginning of the report. Include the following: the client's name, file number, address, phone number, date of birth, age, diagnosis, date of evaluation, name of the evaluator, and the name of the individual who referred the client. If applicable, also note the client's occupation or school level, and parents' names.
2. **Write a statement of the problem.** Describe briefly the client's presenting complaint. To be explicit, write the client's

comments verbatim, and identify them as such in the text. For example: (1) *Mrs. Applegate stated her voice was "scratchy and old sounding."* (2) *Mr. Thomas reported that he stuttered. He said that his "blocked speech" occurred most frequently when he spoke on the telephone.* Note the client's words by using quotation marks. If someone other than the client was the informant, indicate it: *Johnny was accompanied to the clinic by his father, Mr. John Jones, who was the informant during the interview.* Write the diagnostic report in the past tense. You are writing about performance that you observed during the assessment. For example, write: *Joan omitted final consonants in her spontaneous speech.* Do not write *Joan omits final consonants in all her spontaneous speech.* Your observation of the client is limited and your statements must be limited to those observations.

3. **Give background information.** Describe the client's background. Obtain this information from the client's case history, client interview, and reports by other professionals. Give relevant information in detail in this section. Do not report unrelated information that was mentioned. Include the client's developmental history, medical history, social and family history, and educational history in this section. For some clients, it will be necessary to report only certain areas, for other clients, all areas will need to be documented. For example, for a child with language problems, educational background must be described in some detail; but for an adult man with a hoarse voice, detailed educational history may not be necessary. If the reported medical history was unremarkable for speech and language development just say that: *The reported medical history was unremarkable.* However, if a number of illnesses were reported, or if many medications have or are still being prescribed, then carefully document this in the report. Note in this section any previous speech-language pathology services the client has received. Report previous diagnoses. If you summarize information from another professional's report (another speech-language pathologist, a physician, a teacher), always give the professional's name, credentials, and date of report.

4. **Summarize assessment information.** Describe results of the pure-tone audiometric screening, oral peripheral examination, and speech and language assessments.

   Include statements regarding the client's behavior. Include in your **behavioral observations** such information as the client's ability to attend to task and cooperativeness. For example: *The client was cooperative and attended to all tasks with minimal verbal prompting throughout the 1-hour evaluation session. Results were considered representative of the client's abilities.*

You must perform an **audiometric screening** as part of all speech-language evaluations. If it is impossible to perform the screening, note this in the diagnostic report and refer the client for an audiological examination. If a client is wearing hearing aids, perform a hearing aid check before the speech and language assessment to ensure that the hearing aids are operating.

You also must perform an **oral peripheral examination** as part of each diagnostic evaluation. The amount of information that must be written in the report will depend on the results of this examination. If no abnormalities were observed then briefly describe the results. Write in detail any structural or motorical deviations observed.

Describe in detail **the speech and language assessment**. Include information about the client's articulation, voice, fluency, receptive language, and expressive language. You should report results of standardized testing, language sampling, and informal clinical observations of com-municative abilities. Do not just list test scores, say what they mean. For example, a raw score of 9 on the auditory comprehension subtest of the Preschool Language Scale means little to your readers unless they have memorized the test or have the test administration booklet in front of them.

Quantify results of your client's speech sample. Report the total number of words in the sample. When reporting certain behaviors (e.g., correct use of plural /s/), give the percentage of occurrence instead of the specific number of times it was produced. For example: *The client produced the plural /s/ correctly 75% of the obligatory contexts.* This statement is more meaningful than: *The client produced the plural /s/ correctly three times.* If the client omitted specific speech or language structures, give the total number of opportunities (or obligatory contexts) he or she had to produce them. For example: *The client did not produce the plural /s/. The client produced ten phrases that should have contained plural /s/.*

Present the information in a logical and organized sequence. Describe observations relevant to speech, language, voice, fluency, and other aspects in separate paragraphs. Do not confuse the reader by writing about articulation performance in sections describing fluency and voice.

Write a statement about each parameter of speech to suggest that all aspects of the client's speech and language were evaluated, even if no disorder or deviation was exhibited in some areas. For example, if you made no mention of fluency in your report on a child with articulation disorder because you found no problem with it, the reader cannot be sure of this. Therefore, such a statement as, *Analysis of a 200-utterance speech sample revealed 97% fluent speech,* is necessary.

When you present assessment information, do not cross professional boundaries. A common problem occurs when "guessing" at cognitive levels. The speech-language pathologist cannot report I.Q. scores. Neither can you diagnose psychological disorders (depression, mental retardation, and so on). However, you can report behavior that you have observed. For example, you might write: *The client appeared withdrawn throughout the evaluation. That is, he sat with his arms crossed through most of the evaluation and was never observed to make eye contact with the examiner.*

5. **Summarize your impressions.** This section is a summary and interpretation of all the information gathered in your assessment. Report the type and severity of any communicative disorder in this section. Also report if no communicative disorder was exhibited. If a cause for the disorder is known, you may report it in this section. You may make a statement about the prognosis here, or report it in the recommendations section.

6. **Write recommendations.** In this section include the type and amount of service needed, further assessment required, or referral to other professionals. Although specific areas of need should be identified, do not report exact objectives. As you know, additional evaluation, including baselines may need to be performed before starting treatment. You must confer with your clinical supervisor before making specific recommendations.

7. **Sign the report.** Conclude the report with your name, title,

and signature. Your clinical supervisor also will sign the report. Therefore, type his or her name and title. Refer to Appendix J for a sample diagnostic report.

Progress Reports

Progress reports provide information about treatment procedures, the client's performance, and further recommendations. There are several types of progress reports. Two types of commonly used progress reports are described in this section. The first type of progress report is written daily or for every session to document the client's performance. Because they are brief, daily progress reports often are called progress notes. The second type of report is written periodically to summarize the client's progress for a specific treatment period. At the university clinic, the periodic report may be called a Final Summary written at the end of a semester or quarter. Both types of reporting give necessary clinical information.

Daily Progress Notes. You should chart your client's performance in each session. Your practicum site may provide you with a recording form, or you may develop your own. This recording form will include spaces for the client's name, the date of the session, the objective(s), stimuli, client responses, response consequences, and remarks. If you are using unique materials or equipment, you may want to note that on the recording form. A sample treatment recording form is illustrated in Appendix K.

Record the results of each clinical session on a chronological log as soon after the session as possible. This enables you and your supervisor to review the treatment session and make necessary modifications. It also provides a means of communication among professionals. It gives enough information for another clinician to serve your client if you are unable to do so.

One form of charting and reporting client progress is referred to as **SOAP** notes (Flower, 1984). SOAP stands for *subjective, objective, assessment, plan.*

Describe your impressions of the client in the subjective section. For example: *The client appeared very alert and cooperative. He stated, "I'm ready to work hard today."* Write measurable information in the objective section. For instance: *The client produced four syllable phrases with 80% accuracy in 40 out of 50 trials (40/50).*

Describe your analysis of the session in the assessment section. You may also compare the client's performance across sessions in this section. For example: (1) *Production of /r/ increased from 65% accuracy during the last session to 90% accuracy during today's session.* (2) *Withdrawal of visual models resulted in a decrease in accurate production of single syllable words from 90% to 65%.*

Outline the course of treatment in the plan section. You might simply state: (1) *Continue current treatment activities.* (2) *Continue training production of functional CVC words at the imitative level.*

SOAP notes are used more commonly in the medical setting, but may also be used at other practicum sites. If a lesson plan has been prepared in advance of each session, you may sometimes write the results of the session directly on the lesson plan. Because the lesson plan has already detailed the activities, you may just need to note a percentage after an activity. For example: *90% at the word level. 30% at the phrase level.*

Regardless of the form of recording, the data should be accurate and recorded during each session. At the end of the sessions, you may write additional notes. You may make subjective statements, but do not confuse them for observed facts. Also, support your statements with observable data.

Several abbreviations commonly are used in writing progress notes. Refer to Appendix B for some of the commonly used abbreviations. Appendix L contains a sample of progress notes.

Periodic Progress Reports. In medical and private clinics, periodic progress reports are written to summarize a client's treatment and its results. Procedures and their effects on the client's communicative behaviors are described. Again, depending on your practicum assignment, there will be different requirements for writing progress reports. Following is a list of information you will include in most progress reports.

1. Give client identification information. List the client's name, age, address, phone number, occupation or school status, and birthdate. If applicable, give the name of the parent or spouse.
2. Describe the period covered by the report. Note the date the treatment period began and ended. Also note when treatment was originally initiated if different from the beginning period of this report.
3. List the number of sessions attended by the client. You will want to carefully document how many sessions your client

actually attended. You may be reporting on a treatment period covering 3 months in which your client only attended six sessions.

4. List the length of the treatment sessions. You will see clients for differing lengths of time. Some clients may attend 60-minute sessions and others only 30-minute sessions. Include the length of time you spend with your client in each progress report.

5. Briefly summarize the client's status at the beginning of the treatment period. State briefly the client's status before the reporting period. Also, do not write as detailed a description of the client's status at the beginning of the treatment period as you did in your diagnostic report. Give only a brief overview of his or her communicative abilities at the beginning of the treatment period. For example, you might state that, *An analysis of conversational speech in the clinic setting revealed 85% fluency. Analysis of an audiotaped sample of the client's conversational speech at home revealed 82% fluency.*

6. Summarize the treatment plan. Describe the treatment objectives and procedures. Include enough information so the reader will know what your progression of treatment was, and what stimuli and response consequences were used. If the procedure described in the treatment plan was modified, describe the changes and justify them.

7. Describe the client's performance during the period covered by the report. Describe how the client's target behaviors changed during the course of the treatment. Make objective statements such as, *"At the beginning of treatment, Tom's voice was judged hoarse on 90% of his utterances. At the end of the semester, he was judged hoarse on 10% of his utterances."* Include tables and graphs that summarize quantitative data and show changes over the course of treatment.

8. Summarize your conclusions and recommendations. Include in this section your overall impressions of treatment effectiveness. Make a prognostic statement and recommendations based on that prognosis. Did your client make progress? Do you expect your client to continue to make progress? What type of intervention will enable the client to continue to progress? For example: *John demonstrated progress throughout this treatment period. Based on his performance over the past 3 months, prognosis for continued progress is good. It is recommended that John continue to*

receive treatment for his voice disorder. To be most effective, treatment should be given two times per week for a minimum of 30 minutes each session.

9. End your report with your name, title, and signature. Also include your supervisor's name, title, and signature. Refer to Appendix M for a sample progress report.

Final Summaries. At the end of each semester, you must prepare a report for each of the clients you served at the university clinic. This is a report of the client's treatment. The final summary is sometimes interchangeable with a progress report. It contains information similar to a progress report, but often provides more detailed information. As in a progress report, include the following in a final summary.

1. Give client identification information.
2. Identify the period covered by the report.
3. Give the number of sessions attended by the client and the length of the sessions.
4. Summarize the client's status at the beginning of the treatment period.
5. Summarize the treatment plan.
6. Describe the client's performance and improvement.
7. Discuss your conclusions and recommendations.
8. Identify yourself and your supervisor.

See Appendix N for a sample final summary.

Discharge Reports

A discharge report is written for clients dismissed from treatment. Clients are dismissed because they no longer need treatment or do not benefit from it. Others may be dismissed because they do not attend treatment sessions regularly, or have stopped coming to the sessions. Some clients may dismiss themselves from treatment because they cannot afford it.

The discharge report, following a format similar to that of the final summary, covers the treatment period from the beginning of treatment to the discharge date. Sometimes, the differences in reports are more apparent than real. Regardless of the title of the report, a final report is always prepared when a client leaves treatment at any facility. In this case, the discharge report and final summary may be the same.

Record-Keeping Procedures

Besides writing various kinds of reports, student clinicians are responsible for maintaining the client files and an accurate log of their clinical practicum hours. Therefore, you should know the general procedures of maintaining the client records and your practicum records.

Client Files

Clinic records on clients are confidential. Clinic files are kept in a secured area such as a locked room, or in locked file cabinet. You should never leave clinic files unattended in a place where the client's right to confidentiality could be compromised. Never release copies of reports to other professionals or agencies without prior written approval from the client. You are not allowed to take clients' files home.

You are responsible for maintaining your clients' files in a complete and orderly fashion. Follow the procedure established at your clinic for filing documents, recording phone calls, and so on.

To ensure that all necessary information is in their files and is current, review your clients' files periodically. Ask your clients if the phone numbers and addresses in their files are correct. Note all changes in the clients' folders and report them to your clinic secretary.

ASHA's Professional Services Board guidelines (1984) require client records to contain the following information.

1. Client identification information. Telephone number, address, file number, and so forth.
2. The name of the individual or agency that referred the client.
3. Any related information from other agencies, such as copies of medical reports, IEPs, psychological evaluations, and so on.
4. The name of the speech-language pathologist (and student clinician) responsible for service delivery to the client.
5. A diagnostic report. This report may have been performed at another facility.
6. A current treatment plan, including specific objectives and prognosis.

7. Indication of when the treatment plan was discussed with the client or the responsible member of the client's family.
8. Notations regarding conferences held with other professionals.
9. Treatment reports, progress reports, and final summaries.
10. A chronological log of all services provided for the client.
11. Daily progress notes reflecting current status of treatment objectives.
12. A signed and dated consent for release of information.

At the university clinic, the client's file should also contain a signed and dated consent to be observed. All records must be signed by an individual holding current ASHA certification.

Practicum Hours

Student clinicians are responsible for maintaining a log of their clock hours earned in clinical practicum. Your university will provide you with a form for reporting these hours. All clock hours must be verified by a signature of the supervising speech-language pathologist. Chapter 1 describes the activities that may be counted as practicum hours.

Working With Other Professionals

To provide effective services to their clients, speech-language pathologists frequently must work with other professionals. You often will see clients who receive services from such professionals as the physician, physical therapist, psychologist, or special education teacher. You may need to coordinate your services with the service delivered by these professionals. You also must refer clients to other specialists for services. For example, you probably will refer an individual who comes to see you about a voice problem to an otolaryngologist for a laryngeal evaluation. You will refer the individual who does not pass his or her hearing screening to an audiologist for an audiological examination. (Refer to Appendix O for a sample referral letter.) You will consult with professionals in allied health and education professions. To enhance services to clients, speech-language pathologists must develop a working relationship with these professionals.

Roles of Professionals in Allied Services

To work effectively with other professionals, you must know something about their roles. Following is a summary of the services provided by different specialists with whom you may work.

Health Professionals

1. *Audiologist.* The audiologist is a specialist in the identification, measurement, and rehabilitation of hearing impairments. You will work closely with audiologists. For example, you will refer clients who do not pass their hearing screenings to audiologists. You may find that some of your clients have hearing aids that are not functioning correctly. The audiologist may recommend repair, modification, or replacement of the hearing aids. You may work closely with the audiologist in developing a rehabilitation program for a child with a hearing impairment or in developing a program for community access to assistive listening devices. The audiologist is trained to screen for the presence of a speech or language disorder and may refer individuals to you for speech or language services.

2. *Cardiologist.* The cardiologist is a physician with specialized training in cardiovascular diseases (heart disease). Because of the nature of their specialty, cardiologists most frequently work with adults. You may not work frequently with cardiologists, but occasionally you will work with children or adults who have some form of cardiovascular disorder. For example, some of your clients may have a genetic syndrome. Many such syndromes are associated with a high incidence of cardiovascular disorders. Some of the prematurely born infants and children you work with may also have cardiovascular problems. The cardiologist may refer individuals to you who have voice problems because of their reduced lung capacity. You may need to find out from the cardiologist what physical abilities you reasonably can expect from your clients. You also will want to know if medications your clients are taking may affect speech or behavior (e.g., lethargy, attention span, memory).

3. *Neurologist.* The neurologist is a physician with specialized training in function and disorders of the nervous system. Within neurology, there are subspecialties such as pediatric neurology. It is not unusual for the neurologist to work with individuals who also have speech or language disorders. The

neurologist may work with individuals recovering from a cerebrovascular accident (CVA), head trauma, or a variety of other neurological disorders.

The neurologist may request a speech and language assessment of a client recovering from a CVA or head trauma. You must provide detailed information, including prognosis for speech and language development and treatment recommendations.

Your clients with aphasia may be seeing a neurologist or will have seen one. The neurologist can provide information about the extent and location of brain involvement.

Neurologists also work with individuals with behavior disorders. For example, you may be working with a child who begins receiving medication for aggressive behavior. You may need to document any change in speech or language performance after the child takes the medication.

If you work with a client with a seizure disorder, he or she likely will be receiving services from a neurologist. If you suspect a client of having undiagnosed seizures, you may refer the client to a neurologist. You will want to know from all your clients if they are taking medication that may affect their speech, attention span, or alertness.

4. *Occupational therapist.* The registered occupational therapist (OT or OTR), provides evaluation and treatment of daily living skills for individuals with disabilities. This includes assessing and retraining such skills as dressing, cooking, and bathing. The OT also may be involved in training clients in the use of adaptive living devices. Adaptive living devices help individuals live more independently. They include such equipment as modified eating utensils, modified cooking equipment, adaptive equipment for self-dressing, and so on. Your most common interaction with the OT will be in working with patients with dysphagia. Depending on the setting, either the OT or the speech-language pathologist heads the dysphagia team.

   The OT will need to know the patient's communicative abilities. You will provide them with information on the patient's receptive and expressive language. You also will give suggestions on how the OT can help enhance the patient's communicative skills.

5. *Orthodontist.* The orthodontist is a specialist in dental occlusion. You will work closely with the orthodontist providing services for a client with cleft palate, other craniofacial

anomaly, or myofunctional disorder. The orthodontist may request a detailed speech evaluation from you.

6. *Otolaryngologist.* Otolaryngologists are commonly called ENTs —Ear, Nose & Throat specialists. The speech-language pathologist often has a close working relationship with them. You and the otolaryngologist may share such clients as individuals with voice disorders, chronic otitis media, hearing loss, or laryngeal cancer.

If you are working with a child who has a history of chronic otitis media, you should find out what types of medical treatment the child is receiving from the otolaryngologist. You should closely monitor the child's hearing and refer to the physician if there is a decrease in hearing abilities.

If you have a client who has been diagnosed with vocal nodules, the otolaryngologist may consult with you regarding treatment. The otolaryngologist may suggest a trial period of voice treatment before recommending surgical intervention. You carefully will document progress in voice treatment and refer your client back to the otolaryngologist.

You may work with the otolaryngologist in educating the individual facing laryngectomy. After you receive a referral from the otolaryngologist, you will educate the client about communication options following laryngectomy. The laryngologist will inform you of the surgery schedule, and you will meet with the client soon after the surgery to provide an immediate method of communication. You also may arrange for a person who already has had a laryngectomy to meet with your client before and after surgery.

7. *Pediatrician.* The pediatrician is a physician specializing in the medical care of children. You may refer children to their pediatricians because of suspected hearing or vision problems, chronic health problems (allergies, colds, and so on), or unusual behaviors such as poor attention span.

You will encounter pediatricians who are knowledgeable about communicative disorders and many who are not. Unfortunately, a few pediatricians continue to erroneously advise parents that their children will "outgrow" a communication problem. One of your responsibilities is to educate pediatricians about early intervention for speech and language disorders.

8. *Physiatrist.* The physiatrist is a physician with specialized training in rehabilitative medicine. The physiatrist directs the

rehabilitation of a patient who is disabled. Often the disability is caused from CVA or head trauma.

In the medical setting, you may work closely with the physiatrist who may refer patients to you. He or she may request you to give a detailed report on patients' communicative skills, speech and language prognoses, and recommendations.

9. *Physical Therapist.* The registered physical therapist (RPT or PT) provides assessment and treatment for disorders related to physical and musculoskeletal injuries. In the hospital and rehabilitation setting, the speech-language pathologist and physical therapist often provide services for many of the same patients.

   The physical therapist gives you information about patients' motor abilities and optimum positioning and posture for a patient. This information can be essential in developing an appropriate feeding program, or successfully implementing use of an augmentative communication device.

   You will provide the PT with information about patients' communication skills. The PT may want to know what types of instructions (e.g., single word commands) that a patient can understand.

10. *Prosthodontist.* The prosthodontist is a dentist with specialized training in the development and use of prosthetic appliances. The speech-language pathologist and prosthodontist may consult regarding a client with insufficient velopharyngeal closure. You may refer a client with velopharyngeal incompetence to a prosthodontist. A prosthodontist may ask you to help assess velopharyngeal adequacy in a patient before and after a prosthetic appliance is used. You also may be asked for suggestions regarding choice of appliances.

11. *Radiologist.* The radiologist is a physician specializing in the evaluation and treatment of disease with radioactive substances (X-Ray). The radiologist also may perform brain imaging with patients such as those with aphasia. You and the radiologist also may share such patients as those with laryngeal cancer and swallowing disorders.

    Your most frequent contact with the radiologist may involve patients with swallowing disorders. The radiologist may perform videofluoroscopy for patients with dysphagia (swallowing disorders). You may give suggestions regarding positioning of the patient and textures and types of foods to use during the evaluation.

12. *Registered Nurse.* The registered nurse (RN) is responsible for most medical care prescribed by the physician for the patient. Since registered nurses work closely with patients, it is important for the speech-language pathologist and nurse to develop effective communication. The RN can provide information on a patient's daily communicative skills. Another part of patient care is provided by the licensed vocational nurse (LVN) or licensed professional nurse (LPN). The LVN is frequently identified as a nurses aide, has less medical training than the RN, and delivers such care as bathing and feeding patients, and taking vital signs.

    The nursing staff will request information from you on the patient's receptive and expressive abilities. The staff may give you information about communicative attempts of patients. They also may help identify patients needing your services.

13. *Social Worker.* The social worker is often a member of the hospital's rehabilitation team working closely with the patient's family. You can obtain information about community services that your clients may need from the social worker. You also may ask the social worker to intercede with your patients' families who are having difficulty. For example, if you are serving an elderly patient in his or her home, you may observe that neither the spouse nor the patient is able to prepare meals adequately. The social worker may be able to obtain part-time help for the couple or arrange for delivery of meals through social service agencies such as Meals on Wheels.

Educational Specialists

1. *Adaptive Physical Education Specialist.* Adaptive Physical Education Specialists have specialized training in physical education. They have been trained to work with individuals with disabilities. Their services often include providing physical education programs for individuals with disabilities. You probably will not work closely with the adaptive physical education specialist; however, they often are members of the IEP team.

2. *Principal.* School principals are responsible for the day-to-day operations of their schools including the education and well being of all students. The principal can influence the school staff's behaviors and dispositions toward the speech-language pathology program. It is important for you to discuss your

program's goals with the principal. Keep the principal informed regarding such things as the caseload size and types of disorders.

3. *School Nurse.* The school nurse often is responsible for screening students' hearing and vision. The school nurse maintains a health history for each student and often acts as a liaison between the educational staff and other health professionals.

   You will consult regularly with the school nurse about students with hearing loss, voice disorders, and chronic health problems. You may refer students to the school nurse who have poor dentition (such as unrepaired dental caries). You also may refer children with suspected hearing or vision problems to the school nurse.

4. *School Psychologist.* The school psychologist is trained and credentialed to work in the public school setting. The main duties of the school psychologist include testing students to determine their educational strengths and weaknesses. They also determine appropriate educational placement and recommend intervention techniques. The school psychologist may provide some family and student counseling.

   The school psychologist may request you to perform speech and language assessments with some of the students he or she is also evaluating. The school psychologist will ask your opinion regarding how the child's communicative skills may affect educational performance.

   You may need information from the school psychologist about a student's cognitive abilities. You also may ask for help from the school psychologist on managing a child's behavior problems during your treatment sessions.

   It is important for you to establish an effective relationship with school psychologists because they are often the leaders of the IEP team. They can provide support for your program by making appropriate referrals and abiding by your speech and language recommendations.

5. *Special Education Teacher.* The special education teacher is a credentialed teacher with additional training in specific disabilities or disorders. Many students receiving services from a special education teacher also need the services of the speech-language pathologist. Teachers of special education include the following: Teacher of the Hearing Impaired (HI); Teacher of the Learning Handicapped (LH); Teacher of the Severely Emotionally Disturbed (SED); Teacher of the

Orthopedically Handicapped (OH); Teacher of the Severely Handicapped (SH); Teacher of the Visually Impaired (VI); and, Resource Specialist (RS).

You may work with most of these educational specialists. You should develop good communication with these specialists so you can coordinate your services with their services. For example, if the SH teacher is training a child to sit in his or her chair for 5 minutes by using a token reinforcement system, you may follow through with this procedure when you work with the child individually. Conversely, you may be teaching the use of present progressive with a child. You may ask the LH teacher to ask the child to correctly use the present progressive in the classroom setting and reinforce the correct responses.

Guidelines on Establishing Working Relationships With Other Professionals

Regardless of your professional setting, you should be able to communicate effectively with other professionals and obtain all needed services for your client. You should show other professionals that the services you provide are valuable, and that the client needs your services as much as their's. The following are some guidelines that help you accomplish this important task.

1. Provide high quality service at all times so you develop a reputation for excellence.
2. Develop good communication with other professionals. Provide clear, concise, and relevant information. In your reports, describe the effects of your services in direct and measurable terms. Minimize the use of jargon that other professionals may not understand. Provide charts, graphs, and tables when they seem to more clearly show the progress of your clients that just the written narrative.
3. Make sure the clinic sends out assessment and progress reports to those professionals who have referred the client to your clinic. If necessary, talk to the referring professional during the course of the semester to keep them informed about your services.
4. Anytime you discuss a client or your services with other professionals is an opportunity to educate them about speech-

language pathology. Offer accurate information about your services and the needs of particular clients.

5. Respect professional boundaries. Give information only about speech-language pathology. Do not give information, advice, or treatment that is not within the realm of speech-language pathology. Refer the clients to other professional for needed services.

6. Remember that when there is a need to contact another professional, student clinicians must first discuss this with their clinical supervisors to get their advise and approval.

So far, you have learned about various structural and organizational aspects of clinical practicum. You know that you will have opportunities to learn the skills of the profession in a variety of clinical settings. In completing your clinical practicum or internship, you must follow many administrative and ethical rules, regulations, and guidelines.

Once you understand the structures and procedures of clinical practicum, you may concentrate on the clinical methods of speech-language pathology. You will have learned about these methods in various courses taken prior to enrolling in clinical practicum. In the second part of the book, we will give you an overview of these methods that help you treat clients with communicative disorders.

Part II

Clinical Methods in Speech-Language Pathology

I n the Part I of the text, you learned how clinical practicum in speech-language pathology is organized. You also learned some of the rules and guidelines a student clinician must follow.

In Part II, you will find an overview of how to treat adults and children who have various communicative disorders. Selection of target behaviors, treatment procedures to increase desirable communicative behaviors, procedures to decrease undesirable behaviors, and methods to promote maintenance are described.

6

Target Behaviors
Across Disorders

Your starting point for selecting target behaviors depends on what you find out about your clients. You must first find out if the clients assigned to you were assessed or treated at your clinic or have received any kind of clinical services at another clinic.

If the clients have received services at your clinic, you should read carefully the reports in the files. The files may contain an initial assessment (diagnostic) report, treatment reports, progress notes, and reports from other professionals. These reports help you make a rough evaluation of the clients' status.

If the clients were newly referred to the clinic, you should assess them before starting treatment. Assessment procedures were described briefly in chapter 5. Therefore, in this chapter, you will learn about selecting target behaviors for clients of all ages who have many types of communicative disorders.

Selection of Target Behaviors

Most persons with communicative disorders are unable to produce many target behaviors. A child with an articulation disorder, for example, may not produce several phonemes. Another child with a

125

language disorder may not produce many classes of verbal behaviors including grammatic, semantic, or pragmatic features. Similarly, adults with aphasia, people who have had a laryngectomy, persons who are dysarthric, and children with cerebral palsy or hearing loss are unable to produce many target behaviors that are essential for everyday communication. For these and other clients, you need to teach multiple target behaviors.

Though most clients need to learn many target behaviors, they cannot learn them all at once. You select a few behaviors for the initial treatment and continue to teach only a few behaviors at a time. You teach more complex behaviors to clients as they master simpler behaviors. To teach most of the missing communicative behaviors, the clinician must make some initial choices.

The choice is also a matter of sequencing the treatment. You must design a logical sequence of treatment. A sequence is necessary because some behaviors are better taught before other behaviors. Some target behaviors serve an immediate purpose while others must wait until a certain verbal repertoire has been developed. For example, it is better to teach children who are nonverbal such words as *Mommy*, *Daddy*, *juice*, or *car* than it is to teach *red*, *sofa*, or *triangle*. For an adult man with aphasia, it may be better to teach the forgotten name of his wife than it is to teach the name of the local football team in which he never had interest.

Some behaviors *need* to be taught before others. For persons who are nonverbal, it is necessary to teach a basic set of words before teaching word order or other syntactic features. Many morphologic or syntactic features are useless when the child has no basic vocabulary. For example, nouns and verbs need to be taught before many grammatic morphemes can be taught. For example, you cannot teach prepositions (*in*, *on*, *under*) to a child who does not name anything. You cannot teach the auxiliary verb *ing* to a child who does not produce any main verbs (*walk*, *eat*). Similarly, for children who do not produce certain speech sounds, it may be necessary to teach them at the word level before teaching them at the phrase or sentence level. Therefore, the clinician must choose target behaviors at all stages of treatment.

Approaches to Target Behavior Selection

The two main approaches to selecting target behaviors are the normative and the client-specific. In the well established **normative**

approach, you select target behaviors that are appropriate for the client in view of his or her age and the age-based norms. For example, if a 4-year-old child does not produce language behaviors appropriate for 4 year olds, then those behaviors are the targets.

In the more recently developed **client-specific** approach, the targets that make an immediate and significant difference in the client's communication are selected regardless of the norms. In this approach, you do not necessarily follow the table of norms to select target behaviors. You teach behaviors that best serve the client's communicative, educational, and social needs. A study of the client's environment and the educational and social demands made on that client is likely to suggest relevant and useful target behaviors.

In some cases, the normative and the client-specific approaches may suggest the same target behaviors for a given client. However, in many other cases, the targets may be different. The client-specific is more demanding than the normative approach because it requires a greater study of the individual client.

The two approaches contrast more in the case of children than adults and in the case of speech and language targets than other targets. More research is needed to find out the best approach to selecting target behaviors. This means that clinicians cannot automatically assume that norms are the best targets for children. Some evidence suggests that target behaviors that are especially relevant to the client may be better generalized and maintained than those that are selected with no particular regard to the needs of the client (Hegde, 1985). The client-specific approach makes clinical sense because it takes into consideration the uniqueness of each client. Therefore, for the most part, the following guidelines on selecting target behaviors are based on the client-specific strategy.

Guidelines on Selecting Target Behaviors

1. **Select behaviors that will make an immediate and socially significant difference in the communicative skills of the client.** Select target behaviors that will improve the client's social communication, academic achievement, and occupational performance. In treating a child with misarticulations, select those sounds that are most frequently used in conversation and misarticulated by the child *and*

whose correct production will improve intelligibility the most. In treating clients with language disorders, select words that will immediately help the client achieve basic communication. In treating clients with vocal abuse, select the most frequently exhibited abusive behaviors for reduction.

2. **Select the most useful behaviors that may be produced and reinforced at home and in other natural settings.** Such behaviors are likely to be sustained over time. Behaviors that fulfill the needs of the client tend to be produced and reinforced in home and other natural settings. Behaviors that help the client meet the demands made on him or her also tend to be produced and maintained in natural settings.

3. **Select behaviors that help expand the communicative skills.** Teach words that easily may be expanded into phrases and sentences. Though all words can be expanded, some expansions may be more significant to the client than other expansions. For instance, persons who are language impaired who learn such adjectives as *big* and *little* and such nouns as *cup* and *car* can expand them into *big car*, *little cup*, and so forth. Such expansions are more meaningful than what are possible with *triangle* or *refrigerator*.

Potential Target Behaviors Across Disorders

In this section, you will find a range of potential target behaviors that may be appropriate for clients of all ages and disorders of communication. You must remember that the suggested behaviors generally are appropriate, but the final selection depends on an individual client's (a) environment, (b) communicative level before starting treatment, and (c) communicative needs.

Frequent shifts are common in the theory and clinical practice in all areas of speech-language pathology. Therefore, you must read articles in various journals to find out current trends and recent advances in both what to train and how to train. Also, note that student clinicians select target behaviors for their clients only after consulting with their clinical supervisors.

A practical consideration is that each supervisor has his or her views on what to train and how. Since you want to learn different approaches, find out your supervisor's approach. Read the books or articles your supervisor recommends. A more advanced student clinician always can discuss a different approach that she or he wishes to try. Mostly, the student clinician will get the supervisor's approval to try something different. But to first learn what the supervisor has to offer is a good start.

Sometimes, student clinicians wonder whether they should use an approach learned in an academic course which may not agree with what the clinical supervisor recommends. In such cases, discuss the different approaches with the supervisor.

If your supervisor also has taught your academic course on a disorder, make sure you review the class notes and the text used in the class. When you discuss the potential target behaviors for your client with a disorder of articulation, for example, you should review your course information. If it is still current, review the textbook you used. If it is not, read a more recently published book on articulation and phonology. When you discuss your client with your supervisor, you should be knowledgeable about the disorder under discussion.

Articulation and Phonological Disorders

The first few clients assigned to most undergraduate student clinicians may have articulation or language disorders. This is because in the typical undergraduate academic sequence, courses on articulation disorders and language disorders are likely to precede courses on other communicative disorders. Therefore, the very first client you treat may have a disorder of articulation or language. We, therefore, will start with articulation and phonological disorders.

Obviously, a client with an articulation disorder does not produce or only inconsistently produces certain speech sounds. Equally obvious is that the treatment targets are those sounds that are not produced correctly. However, as you have found out from your academic courses, the nature of articulation disorders makes the process of selecting treatment targets a bit more complicated.

Most of the complications are due to theoretical shifts in the study of articulation and its disorders. Because of changing theories, the treatment targets for clients with articulation disorders have changed dramatically over the past few years, although some fundamentals have remained the same. Some of the changes may not be as substantial as they initially appear, but shifts in theories have suggested apparently dissimilar treatment targets for clients with articulation disorders. Student clinicians need to learn different approaches that are supported by clinical data. Therefore, the major approaches to selecting articulatory target behaviors are summarized here.

An overview of assessment of articulation was described in chapter 5. It was pointed out there that an analysis of your assessment or reassessment data will show the types and variety of speech sound errors made by the client. You summarize the number of sounds in error, the frequency of those errors, and the types of errors. Further analysis may be made of the patterns of errors. The pattern analysis may depend either on distinctive feature theory or phonological theory. This analysis sets the stage for selecting treatment targets.

Selection of Individual Sounds for Training. Most experts agree that a mild disorder of articulation does not require a pattern analysis. Patterns may be discovered when the child misarticulates many phonemes forming classes of misarticulations that are handled more efficiently as error groups. When this is not the case, the traditional sound-by-sound approach will be adequate.

Select individual sounds for training when one or more of the following conditions are met.

- The child's speech is generally intelligible.
- Only a few sounds are in error.
- The errors of articulation are due to such organic factors as cleft palate, velopharyngeal insufficiency, and neurological involvement.

The meaning of *only a few sounds in error* is not always precise. The critical point is that the phonemes in error do not form significant patterns based on distinctive features or phonological processes. A few errors, even if they share distinctive features, may be handled efficiently within the sound-by-sound approach. Patterns or relations are unlikely in case of just a few misarticulations. Also, the analysis of a negligible pattern that may underlie misarticulations of a few phonemes may not add much to treatment economy or efficiency.

Use the sound-by-sound analysis to determine target behaviors in the following manner.

1. Find out if each phoneme is produced correctly or not.
2. Classify errors as either substitutions, distortions, or omissions.
3. Find out the word positions in which the sounds are misarticulated.

4. Select the initial target sounds for training and write your target behavior statements in objective and quantitative terms.

The following is an example of a target behavior statement for a child who substitutes /w/ for /r/ in all word positions:

The target is the correct production of /r/ at 90% accuracy in conversational speech produced at the clinic and the child's home. The correct productions should be observed in all word positions and in at least three consecutive speech samples each containing a minimum of 20 opportunities for producing the target phoneme.

Note that the example of target behavior description specifies:

1. a quantitative criterion of performance (90% correct);
2. the response mode (conversational speech);
3. the response setting (clinic and the child's home);
4. the number of speech samples in which the target behavior productions are documented (three samples); and
5. the number of opportunities for producing the target phoneme in each sample (20).

The quantitative criteria mentioned in the example of target behavior description are only suggestive. Each of those criteria may be modified. A different response setting may be specified. For example, depending on the client, classrooms or work places may be the settings in which the target phoneme productions are documented. Discuss these criteria with your clinical supervisor who may suggest alternatives.

In writing target behavior statements, avoid such phrases as "the client will produce /s/ in conversational speech." Whether the target behavior will be learned or not will depend on many variables. Also, state when the client will meet the goal in probabilistic terms, not by a certain date. It is acceptable to make such probabilistic statements as "the phoneme (or phonemes) are expected to be learned in 3 months of therapy given twice weekly in 30-minute sessions."

Selection of Sound Patterns for Treatment. Theories of normal and disordered sound production have described several patterns, clusters, or classes. When a theory describes patterns of misarticulations, the treatment goal is their elimination. When a theory describes patterns of normal sound production, then the treatment goal is to teach the missing patterns to a client. Three patterns are available for selection: (1) patterns based on place-manner-voice analysis, (2) patterns based on distinctive features, and (3) patterns based on phonological processes.

Patterns Based on Place-Manner-Voice Analysis. This older method of classifying speech sounds into patterns is based on how they are produced normally. In the place-manner-voice analysis, errors of substitution are classified according to similarities in the place of articulation, manner of articulation, or in the presence or absence of voicing. In this method, you find patterns in multiple substitutions that are based on the place or manner of articulation or the feature of voicing.

You can find patterns based on place-manner-voicing in the following manner.

1. Find out all substitution errors of the client.
2. Group those substitutions that are based on place of articulation. For instance, a child may substitute lingua-alveolars for linguadentals (e.g., d/ð; or linguavelars may be substituted for lingua-alveolars (e.g., k/t; g/d).
3. Group those substitutions that are based on manner of production. Sounds produced in one manner may be substituted for sounds produced in another manner. For instance, a child may substitute stops for fricatives (e.g., b/v; t/s; p/f) and glides for liquids (e.g., w/r; w/l)
4. Group those substitutions that are based on voicing feature. A child, for instance, may substitute voiced sounds for voiceless sounds (e.g., b/f; g/k).
5. Teach one or more sounds from each group. Probe to find out if untrained sounds in the group are produced without training (generalization). For example, teach a few fricatives to a child who substitutes stops for fricatives; teach a few voiceless sounds to a child who uses voiced sounds instead. Find out if the untrained fricatives or untrained voiceless sounds are produced. If not, teach them as well. Generalization may or may not occur; if it does, you will save clinical training time. Still, you should extend treatment to nonclinical settings for maintenance.

See chapter 7 for training procedures. How to probe for generalization also is described in that chapter.

The following is an example of a target behavior description for a client who substitutes voiced sounds for voiceless sounds:

> The target is the correct production of voiceless sounds [specify them] in all word positions at 90% accuracy in conversational speech evoked at the clinic and at the child's home. The correct productions should be observed in at least three consecutive speech samples. Each speech sample should have at least 20 opportunities for producing the target phoneme.

When you write a target behavior statement for a pattern of misarticulation, you must **list the individual sounds** as well. Just saying that you will teach voiced sounds or fricatives will not be specific enough. It is likely that not all sounds in a category are in error. Even if they are, you do not teach a category or a pattern directly. You teach concrete individual sounds that belong to a conceptual category or pattern.

Patterns Based on Distinctive Features. In the 1970s, the distinctive feature approach to articulation training was researched frequently. Though researched less frequently in recent years, you may wish to learn this approach by using it with a client or two. As you know, distinctive features are unique characteristics that distinguish one speech sound from the other. A feature system proposed by Chomsky and Halle (1968) has been used widely. Using a binary system of pluses and minuses, Chomsky and Halle have described 11 distinctive features of English consonants.

The distinctive feature analysis is not much different from the traditional place-manner-voice analysis (Elbert & Gierut, 1986). What is new about it—the binary system—is only a superficial application of a quantitative method with very little mathematical meaning. However, clinical training is the only way to test the validity of distinctive features. If they are valid, untrained sounds with the same features as the trained sounds should be produced on the basis of generalization. Therefore, you can do some informal clinical experimentation while using this approach. A client who is trained on a few sounds that share a set of features should begin to produce other missing sounds that have the same features without training. Reliable baselines and continuous treatment data will help you determine if this happens in treatment.

Take the following steps in using distinctive features to find patterns of misarticulations.

1. Find out all the errors of your client.
2. Determine the distinctive features shared by the phonemes in error.
3. Group misarticulated sounds on the basis of shared (common) distinctive features.
4. Teach a few sounds from each group. Probe to see if untrained sounds within the group are produced without training. If they do, reinforce them and implement a maintenance procedure.

The following is an example of a target behavior description for a client who substitutes nonnasal sounds for nasal sounds (d/n; b/m; g/ŋ). The assumption is that the client has not mastered the distinctive feature *nasal* or has not mastered the contrast between nasal and nonnasal sounds.

> The target is the correct production of nasal sounds (/n/, /m/, and /ŋ/) in all word positions at 90% accuracy in conversational speech evoked at the clinic and at the child's home. The correct productions should be observed in at least three consecutive speech samples. Each speech sample should have at least 20 opportunities for producing the target phoneme.

Note, again, that you should specify the sounds that are taught. Do not write "stridency will be taught." Instead, list the sounds that share the feature stridency. You cannot teach a distinctive feature directly. You only can teach some sounds that have certain features. The value of the method, as pointed out, is in monitoring potential production of untrained sounds. The system simply makes it easier to track the effects of treating some sounds on other, untrained sounds.

Patterns Based on Phonological Processes. Most experts now recommend a phonological approach to organize target behaviors for persons with multiple misarticulations resulting in limited speech intelligibility (Bernthal & Bankson, 1988; Hodson, 1980; Stoel-Gammon & Dunn, 1985). There are several phonological process analyses that are not totally compatible. Ultimately, your systematic clinical work will help you select the one that has worked the best. Eventually, you may modify an approach in light of your experience and use it consistently. Meanwhile, clinical research may show that a particular approach is better than others. During your clinical practicum, you may experiment with different approaches or use the one suggested by your supervisor.

You should know the basic phonological processes to select the appropriate processes for a given client. Though there is no full agreement among experts on the total number of processes, the following are most frequently described in the literature and are categorized as shown (Bernthal & Bankson, 1988; Stoel-Gammon & Dunn, 1985).

Frequently used phonological processes are:

I. **Syllable Structure Processes.** In these processes, the structure of syllables is changed.

   Final Consonant Deletion. Certain final consonants are omitted.

   [ba] for ball; [da] for Daddy.

   Unstressed Syllable Deletion. An unstressed initial or medial syllable is omitted.

   [medo for tomato]; [tɛfon] for telephone

   Reduplication. A syllable, part of a syllable, or a monosyllabic word is repeated.

   [wawa] for water; [gogo] for go.

   Epenthesis. Addition of an unstressed sound, often the vowel [ə].

   [bəlak] for black; [bigə] for big.

   Cluster Reduction. Most frequently, omission of a sound in a cluster of sounds; sometimes, one of the sounds of a cluster may be deleted and another may be substituted.

   [bu] for blue; [cod] for cold;
   [no] for [snow]; [fi] for tree.

II. **Substitution Processes.** In these processes, target sounds are replaced by other sounds. These processes often involve changes based on place of articulation or manner of articulation.

The following two processes are based on a shift in place of articulation.

Fronting. A sound typically produced in the back is replaced by the one produced in the front of the oral cavity.

[ti] for key; [su] for shoe.

Backing. A sound typically produced in the front is replaced by the one produced in the back of the oral cavity.

[gu] for do; [kæn] for tan.

The following processes are based on a shift in the manner of articulation.

Gliding of Liquids. A glide is produced instead of a liquid; observed also in consonant clusters.

[wʌn] for run; [bwo] for blow.

Stopping. A stops is produced instead of a fricative or an affricate.

[tʌn] for sun; [du] for zoo.

Affrication. An affricate is produced instead of a fricative.

[tʃu] for shoe; [tʃn] for sun.

Deaffrication. Affricates are replaced by sounds of other kind.

[sap] for chop; [dʌmp] for jump.

Vocalization. A vowel, typically [o] or [u] is produced instead of a syllabic liquid.

[nudu] for noodle; [zipu] for zipper.

Denasalization. A nonnasal sound is produced instead of a nasal sound (the manner of production may be similar for the target and the substituted sound).

[bud] for moon; [deis] for nice.

Glottal Replacements. The glottal stop is produced instead of a sound in the final or intervocalic position.

[baʔl] for bottle; [tuʔ] for tooth.

III. **Assimilation Processes.** In these processes, one sound becomes more like another sound. In progressive assimilation, a sound is assimilated to a previous sound as in [bup] for boot; in regressive assimilation, a sound is assimilated to a subsequent sound, as in [b mp] for jump. Several kinds of assimilation processes are described:

Velar Assimilation. A nonvelar sound changes into a velar sound.

[kok] for coat (progressive);
[kek] for take (regressive).

Nasal Assimilation. A nonnasal sound changes into a nasal sound.

[mʌni] for bunny; [nʌn] for done.

Labial Assimilation. A nonlabial sound changes into a labial sound.

[pip] for pit; [bup] for boot.

Prevocalic Voicing. A voiceless consonant in prevocalic positions is voiced.

[dam] for Tom; [bep] for paper.

Devoicing of Final Consonants. A voiced consonant in final word positions is devoiced.

[bæk] for bag; [nos] for nose.

IV. Metathesis is an additional phonological process in which   sounds are transposed.

>   [ɛfəlʌnt] for elephant.
>   [æmələn] for animal.
>   [bæksɪt] for basket.

In learning to use a phonological approach in analyzing multiple misarticulations, take the following steps.

1. Select one phonological analysis procedure as there are several somewhat incompatible approaches.
2. Following the procedure prescribed by the selected approach, record continuous speech samples, transcribe the samples, and make a process analysis.
3. Select processes for intervention. Remember, you teach specific sounds to eliminate a process.

Most experts recommend that your initial targets should be those processes that (1) reduce intelligibility the most, (2) include sounds from different classes, (3) are outgrown sooner by normally developing children, and (4) tend to persist in children with multiple misarticulations.

When you have selected a process for remediation, write target behavior descriptions that specify what sounds will be taught. Do not simply state that the "goal of treatment is to eliminate final consonant deletion." It is both abstract and negative. Also, the reader would not know what you do to eliminate a process. Instead, specify the process to be eliminated and the sounds to be taught:

> The treatment goal is to eliminate the final consonant deletion process by teaching the correct production of the following consonants in word final positions: [list the phonemes]. The final criterion is at least 90% accuracy in the production of the target phonemes in three conversational speech samples recorded in nonclinical settings.

Note that no phonological process is eliminated without training certain individual phonemes. Phonological processes are theoretical ways of grouping errors; they should not be confused with treatment methods.

Language Disorders

What to teach children with language problems was controversial during the times when theories of language were changing rapidly.

When speech-language pathologists began to study Chomsky's transformational generative grammar in the 1960s and 1970s, other language targets seemed inappropriate. Some years later, when the semantic theory of language became popular, teaching vocabulary or grammar was considered a dated practice. Finally, when the pragmatic theory was hailed as the latest revolution in the study of language, teaching anything other than pragmatic rules was considered passé.

Though theoretical advances continue, the magnitude of theoretical shifts has diminished. While we are always looking over our shoulders for that next revolution, we have learned in recent years that new theories did not eliminate the need to teach what the old theory said we should. New theories only listed additional behaviors to teach. Obviously, it would be foolish to claim that we do not have to teach vocabulary or grammatical morphemes or syntactical features just because of an emphasis on pragmatics of language. Because pragmatics concerns the use of language, a child or an adult who does not produce words, phrases, and sentences at all has no use for pragmatics. You cannot use what you do not have. Clinically, pragmatic concerns are especially important at an advanced stage in therapy. Having established certain language behaviors, you promote their naturalistic production (McCormick & Schiefelbusch, 1990; Owens, 1991; Reed, 1986; Schiefelbusch & Lloyd, 1988; Warren & Rogers-Warren, 1985;).

In treating most if not all disorders of communication, you shape the final target behaviors from simpler behaviors. Clinicians continuously build more complex behaviors by integrating simpler ones. This is especially true of language because it is the most integrative of all communicative behaviors. We build this abstract, integrative structure by teaching simpler, concrete responses.

Student clinicians need not wonder about the final target behavior for people who are language impaired. It is always the same: personally significant and socially useful verbal skills. This final target often is theoretical and sometimes not achieved. Each client reaches a certain level of proficiency in learning those skills. But there is no question that we would like to take clients who are language impaired to the highest level of performance that can be achieved with the best possible techniques.

Student clinicians often wonder about the starting point. A general rule that applies to all clients is that it depends on the client. The initial selection of targets depends mostly on the existing language repertoire of the client. This is true of children and adults with language problems that may have varied etiology or associated conditions. In many children, the diagnosis may be language delay or disorder. In other children and most adult clients, it may be a language disorder associated with neurological disease or damage. In clients of any age, language disorder may be associated with mental retardation, autism, hearing impairment, physical disabilities, or other conditions. In each case, you should find out the client's communicative repertoire and build on it. A careful analysis of your assessment data will help you select the initial target behaviors.

Language Targets I. Basic Vocabulary. To many infants and children with language delay, the initial verbal targets are a set of words. Although you should not select some standard set of canned target words for each client, you can use a few general guidelines to select words that give a good starting point for language treatment. For instance, select.

1. **Concrete words that name specific things or actions.** For the initial targets, do not select generic or abstract words. For instance, do not try to teach such words as *toys, food* or *clothes*. Instead teach specific words like *car, milk*, and *sock*.
2. **Names (nouns) of manipulable objects.** Teach names of toys (*car, truck, ball, balloon, train, choo choo*) the child plays with. Also, teach words that name food items (*milk, juice, cookie*) clothing and personal belongings (*shirt, sock, shoe, hat*) names of family members (*brother, sister, mommy, daddy, grandma, grandpa*).
3. **Names of animals and pets.** Teach these names and later integrate them into short stories to expand the vocabulary and to teach sentence structures.
4. **Verbs.** Select commonly used verbs (*run, jump, hop, walk, push, laugh, smile, eat, drink*). Represent them by action that might help keep the child's interest in therapy. Once taught, use the verbs to teach basic sentence structures.
5. **Adjectives to describe objects and people.** Teach simple adjectives (*big, small, tall, short, red, green*) that can be used later to expand the client's utterances.

Language Targets II. Phrases. Teach phrases when the child can produce several single words. Initially, teach two-word phrases. As the child learns more phrases, increase the number of words in utterances until the child is ready to learn morphological and syntactic elements of language. For example, use.

1. **Simple phrases.** Combine already learned words to form the initial target phrases to teach. For example, teach two-word

utterances that are a combination of adjectives and nouns the child reliably produces (*big ball, little car, red sock*).

2. **Two-word utterances that are a combination of nouns and action verbs.** You may teach such phrases as *boy run, kitty jump, baby eat.*

3. **Two- or three-word utterances.** Form these by combining already learned and yet to be learned words. Requests or mands are excellent for this kind of target responses. For example, teach such combinations as *want milk, more juice, cookie, please*, and so forth. Other targets may include nouns and verbs: *ball hit, boy hit ball*, and *push car.*

Language Targets III. Morphological and Syntactic Elements. Start morphological training when a child can produce phrases. While teaching morphological elements, you may continue to teach new words and multi-word phrases to expand the child's verbal repertoire. Before you can teach syntactic structures, you need to teach the following (and several other) grammatical morphemes.

1. **Morphological features that help build a language repertoire.** See what features may be integrated into the existing language responses. You know the selected responses should be useful to the individual child so they are likely to be produced and reinforced at home.

2. **The present progressive** *ing.* This is one of the early morphological features to teach. Use the already taught noun and verb combinations to teach the use of the present progressive. For example, you could teach *boy running, Daddy coming, frog jumping, kitty eating* and so forth.

3. **Prepositions** (*car in box, book on table*), **regular plurals** (*two cups, my cookies, give me marbles*), **possessives** (*Daddy's hat, Mommy's coat, Kitty's tail*), **articles** (*I want a cookie, give me the ball*), **regular past tense inflections** (*I missed it, he jumped, she smiled*), and **irregular past tense words** (*he went, I ate, she broke*).

4. **Morphological features that help expand the multiword utterances into syntactically more correct utterances or complete sentences.** Expand the previously taught phrases into longer utterances by adding additional grammatical features. For example, by adding the auxiliary verb *is*, you can expand the multiword utterances into such sentences as *the boy is running, the man is working, the girl is smiling* and

so forth. Copula will also help expand phrases into sentences (*The man is nice, the lady is beautiful, the dog is big, the cat is small*). Expand phrases used to teach prepositions into sentences (*car is in the box, book is on the table*).

5. **Pronouns.** Teach them by using other, already taught sentence structures (*she is walking, he is eating, it is coming; this is my coat, that is your hat*).

6. **Other grammatical morphemes and syntactic structures.** Select those that help form complex forms of sentences. For example, teach questions involving *who, what, where, why, how, and when*. Also, teach negative sentences involving *no, not, nothing* and so forth.

Language Targets IV. Functional Units and their Social Use. So far, we have described various structural elements of language that are appropriate for early and intermediate training. In the more advanced stages of language treatment, broader, functional or pragmatic units may be taught. Always remember that the final goal of language intervention is to promote appropriate conversational speech in natural settings.

In speech-language pathology, functional units have two different meanings. In pragmatics, functional units mean language structures that have different speaker intentions and listener effects. Sometimes also called speech acts, functional units may express needs or feelings, control other persons, establish communication, and so forth. Other functional units include utterances that call for attention, request information, give information, request action, and respond to requests. Pragmatic structures especially relevant to conversational speech include topic initiation, topic maintenance, turn taking, and conversational repair (James, 1990; Owens, 1988, 1991). As you can see, pragmatic (functional) units are not based on the structure of language as morphologic or syntactic units are. Instead, they are based on what they do for both the speaker and the listener.

Functional units that have a different meaning are described in the behavioral analysis of language. Like pragmatics, behavioral analysis also describes language in functional units. These units are not based on the structure of language. The difference between the behavioral and pragmatic units of language is that the behavioral units are based on a cause-effect analysis. That is, verbal behaviors are divided into different groups because the responses belonging to those groups have different causes. In a general sense, this is what pragmatic units are supposed to be, but may or may not be. From the very beginning, behavioral analysis has emphasized functional units as against structural units of language. Though initially rejected by both linguists and speech-language pathologists alike, the basic logic of the behavioral analysis is now being appreciated, especially in language intervention (Warren & Rogers-Warren, 1985).

The basic logic of the behavioral analysis is that meaningful units of language are not structures but cause-effect (functional) units that describe what a speaker said, why it was said, and what effects it had on the listener (Skinner, 1957; Winokur, 1976). Therefore, a functional unit specifies not just an utterance, but the circumstance under which it is produced and the effects that follow. A functional unit of verbal behavior is defined as a causal relation between an utterance, its antecedent, and its consequence. The utterance may be described structurally; it may be a word, a phrase, a sentence and so on. The antecedent may be either an event in the environment or an internal, typically motivating state of the speaker (hunger or pain, for instance). The consequence is the effect the utterance has on a listener or listeners.

Though there are important differences between them, both pragmatics and behavioral analysis have drawn attention to meaningful units of speech as they are produced in specified conditions to produce specified effects. If speech is useful, it is precisely because it affects the behavior of other persons. Language is a tool only in this sense: you can accomplish something with it. Language-disordered children lack that powerful social tool. Therefore, in language intervention, you eventually must teach conversational skills that give such children a means to express themselves and to affect others.

Research continues to be done on teaching behavioral and pragmatic functional units. These units will be refined as clinical data emerge. Also, you will find new targets as researchers describe and evaluate them. Meanwhile, consider teaching the following pragmatic language categories.

1. **Requests or mands.** In pragmatics, requests are subdivided into requests for action, information, objects, and so on. In the behavioral analysis, all requests, commands, demands, and similar utterances are classified into a single functional response unit called mands. It is possible that when a client learns to make certain kinds of requests, other kinds of requests will be made without further training. Obviously, this can happen only when the client produces the basic words to

make any kind of request. If not, you must first teach selected words. As you do with any other response category, teach one or two types of requests or mands and probe to see if the client begins to produce other kinds of requests or mands.

2. **Tacts or descriptive statements.** Children and adults with limited language do not readily describe or talk about events in their environment. They may not comment on things and objects that evoke speech from most people. Statements that describe and comment on things, events, and persons are called tacts in the behavioral analysis. Such statements are excellent pragmatic targets to teach. In teaching them, you should often include such other conversational skills as described next.

3. **Topic initiation.** This skill is emphasized in pragmatic research. Persons who are language impaired do not readily start talking about a topic. Technically, topic initiation requires that the speaker be the first one to introduce a new topic for conversation. However, with most clients who are language impaired, you will have to say something to have the child begin conversation on a topic. For example, you may have to ask questions on a topic to prompt the client to begin talking.

4. **Topic maintenance.** Once the client begins to initiate conversation, topic maintenance becomes an appropriate target to teach. Again, persons who are language impaired tend not to stay on a topic of conversation. They may shift from one topic to another without saying much on any of them. To overcome this problem, you can target progressively longer durations of speech on targeted topics of conversation.

5. **Turn taking in conversation.** Conversational speech requires that two or more individuals take turn in speaking and listening. Each person engaged in conversation is both a speaker and a listener. A person who plays only one of these roles is not a good conversational partner. Therefore, it is necessary to teach the language impaired to talk and to listen in an alternating manner.

6. **Conversational repair.** This is another conversational skill described in pragmatics. Many persons who are language impaired fail to do something when they do not understand what is said to them. This may be a reason why they do not continue conversation. Normally, the listener who does not understand a speaker suggests this in some way to the speaker. The listener may say "tell me more about it," "I don't understand," "please speak louder," and so forth. Such statements

prompt the speaker to simplify, change words, expand, and repeat to modify the utterance in these and many other ways. Both the listener actions and the speaker modifications are involved in conversational repair. Teach clients to request more information, ask for clarification, or to say "I don't understand."

7. **Narration.** A more complex language skill is to narrate events, stories, and experiences in a cohesive and chronologically correct manner. Obviously, before you target narrative skills, you must have taught many other skills including vocabulary, morphologic features, and syntactic aspects of language.

Voice Disorders

Voice disorders include many kinds of problems. Some are related to abnormal vocal fold actions, others to oral and nasal resonance, several to physical diseases, and many to general behaviors of the client that have an impact on the health of the vocal folds. After a medical examination and a careful voice assessment, you determine the nature of the disorder and the target behaviors to be trained to eliminate that disorder (Boone & McFarlane, 1988; Wilson, 1987).

Target Behaviors in Disorders of Phonation. Some disorders of phonation are due to physical problems or diseases. Among these are paralysis and ankylosis, carcinoma, varieties of laryngeal tumors and lesions, infections, and papilloma. Other disorders of phonation are due to abuse or misuse of the vocal mechanism.

In treating disorders of phonation that have physical causes, the necessary medical or surgical treatment is carried out first. Then the voice therapy techniques are used to improve the functioning of the vocal mechanism. When surgery removes the laryngeal structures as in laryngectomy, you should integrate new ways of phonation or new sources of phonation into the voice therapy. In treating disorders of phonation due to vocal abuse or misuse, you must change the vocal and general behavior of the client. Because a majority of voice disorders are related to vocal abuse or misuse, a major task of the voice clinician is to change vocally abusive behaviors and to modify patterns of misuse.

Some of the typical behaviors targeted in treating disorders of phonation include the following.

1. **Respiration training.** Use this target when there is evidence of faulty use of the airstream during phonation and continuous speech. A specific target is a deep enough inhalation to sustain utterances of typical length. Sustained exhalation while prolonging certain vowels is a common target.

2. **Muscular effort.** Some patients have difficulty in approximating their vocal folds because of unilateral cord paralysis, general fatigue, and myasthenia. Such patients need to exert muscular effort in achieving vocal cord approximations. A specific target is to teach the client to push on the arm of the chair on which he or she is sitting and phonate simultaneously. Hard glottal attacks also have been targeted in such cases.

3. **Esophageal speech.** This is a target for patients who have undergone laryngectomy. In teaching esophageal speech, target either the injection or inhalation of air; in some cases, the two may be combined. In injecting air into the esophagus, the patient is asked to first impound some air in the oral cavity and then push it back. The production of plosive consonants especially are helpful in this process. In inhaling air into the esophagus, the patient rapidly takes in air while keeping the esophagus relaxed and open. The air passing through the esophagus produces vibrating sound which is articulated into speech sounds.

4. **Phonation with artificial larynx.** An alternative target for the laryngectomee, phonation with artificial larynx involves the use of mechanical devices to produce sound that is articulated into speech sounds.

5. **Relaxation.** When there is evidence of excessive muscular tension affecting the voice of the patient, muscular relaxation might be a useful target. Systematic relaxation of specific muscle groups is targeted.

6. **Vocal rest.** This is a target for patients with infectious or traumatic laryngitis. The patient is asked to refrain from speaking and whispering.

7. **Altered head positions.** Changing the head position while speaking often results in better voice. You must try different head positions to find a position that promotes better voice quality. Extended, flexed, or tilted head positions have all been noted to change the voice.

8. **Elimination of vocally abusive behaviors.** Target the following for reduction.

(a) Yelling and screaming
(b) Smoking
(c) Coughing and frequent throat clearing
(d) Excessive talking, singing, crying, or laughing
(e) Talking too much with allergic reactions and upper respiratory infection
(f) Talking in noisy situations

9. **Elimination of vocal misuse.** Reduce the following:
   (a) Frequent use of hard glottal attack
   (b) Excessively loud speaking
   (c) Habitual speaking with inappropriate pitch levels
   (d) Continuous speaking or singing for extended durations

Target Behaviors in Disorders of Loudness and Pitch. The term disorders of loudness and pitch is self-explanatory. Disorders of loudness include both excessive loudness or insufficient loudness of voice. Disorders of pitch include too high or too low a pitch for a given person.

The following target behaviors are appropriate in treating disorders of pitch; remember, each target is client specific.

1. **Increased loudness.** This is a target for clients who speak excessively softly. Select a client-specific level of loudness.
2. **Decreased loudness.** This is a target for those who speak with excessive loudness. Again, select loudness level that is appropriate for the client.
3. **Higher pitch.** In the typical case of high-pitched male voice, target a client-specific lower pitch.
4. **Lower pitch.** In the low-pitched female voice, target a higher pitch. The target pitch is relative to the client's typical pretreatment pitch.

Target Behaviors in Disorders of Resonance. Disorders of resonance include hypernasality, hyponasality, and reduced oral resonance. The clinical targets are obvious and include the following.

1. **Reduced nasal resonance on non-nasal speech sounds.** This is a target for many clients including those with hearing impairment, velopharyngeal incompetence, cleft palate, and paralysis of the velum associated with cerebral palsy, stroke, and other neurological problems. A predominant voice problem in these clients is hypernasality.

2. **Increased nasal resonance on nasal speech sounds.** This is a target for clients with hyponasality (denasality). People who are hearing impaired, among others, may need this target.
3. **Increased oral resonance.** In some cases of resonance disorders, lack of oral resonance is a dominant problem. In them, you increase oral resonance.

Disorders of Fluency

Apparently, disorders of fluency are treated in many different ways. Historically, the targets in stuttering treatment programs have varied because of varied definitions of stuttering. Among other targets, increased self-confidence, reduced anxiety, resolution of social role conflict, reduction of parental concern for normal nonfluencies, improved self-image, fluent stuttering, acceptance of stuttering, modification of negative attitudes, and resolution of repressed psychological conflicts have all been targeted. That these targets may not be appropriate is suggested by lack of documented evidence for their effectiveness in reducing stuttering (Bloodstein, 1987; Hegde, 1985; Ingham, 1984).

In recent years, many effective treatment programs have been researched. Though different treatment packages differ somewhat from each other, almost all of them use some or all of the following targets.

1. **Management of airflow.** This target behavior has two components. The first is a slightly exaggerated inhalation of air. The second is a slight exhalation of air through the mouth before starting phonation. Make sure the client does not impound the air in the lungs. A small amount of air must be exhaled as soon as the peak of inhalation is reached. You may use this target with most stutterers, but especially with those whose stutterings are associated with mismanaged airflow.
2. **Gentle onset of phonation.** Teach the client to initiate phonation gently after the slight exhalation of air through the mouth. The phonatory onset should be relaxed, soft, and easy.
3. **Reduced rate of speech through syllable prolongation.** Reduce the rate of speech to a level where speech is free from stuttering. Note that the initial target speech rate is client-specific. Some have to slow down more than others to

maintain a stutter-free speech. Do not reduce the rate by pauses between words or phrases; reduce it by syllable (mostly vowel) prolongation. Teach the production of phrases and sentences without gaps between words. The client should produce words as though they were a string of prolonged syllables without word boundaries.

4. **Normal prosody.** The rate reduction and explicit management of airflow and phonatory onset result in an unnatural fluency. Therefore, in the final stages of treatment, shape normal prosody including a near-normal rate, intonation, and rhythm.

5. **Maintenance of fluent conversational speech in natural settings.** This is the final target. Make sure that at the time of dismissal, the client is around 98% fluent in the clinic. This high rate of fluency is not expected to be maintained in the natural settings. A minimum of 95% fluency must be maintained over time.

In the treatment of cluttering, another disorder of fluency, reduced rate and more deliberate articulation of speech sounds have been targeted. Teaching maintenance of intelligible and fluent speech in clutterers is still a major clinical challenge.

Neurogenic Communicative Disorders in Adults

Several types of communicative disorders are associated with neurological disease or damage. These disorders include aphasia, apraxia, and dysarthria.

Though some form of neurological condition is associated with these disorders of communication, the patients in this general group are highly varied. There are subgroups within each diagnostic category. Individual differences in subgroups are also significant as they are in all groups of persons with (or without) communicative problems. Therefore, a comprehensive description of target behaviors for adults and children with neurogenic communicative disorders is beyond the scope of this book. There are several excellent sources that you should read carefully (Boone, 1972; Davis, 1983; Johns, 1985; Rosenbeck, LaPointe, & Wertz, 1989; Yorkston, Beukelman, & Bell, 1988).

Target Behaviors for Aphasic Patients. Aphasia is an impairment in understanding, formulating, and expressing language due to brain damage. Before selecting target behaviors, the complex pattern of neurological and verbal deficits must be evaluated carefully. The individual patient's pattern of deficits will determine the selection of target behaviors. Select them only after a careful assessment of the type of aphasia, the patient's predominant problems, his or her communicative needs, and chances of some immediate success at communication. Make sure the selected behaviors are meaningful and pragmatic for the patient.

Some of the commonly suggested target behaviors for many aphasic patients include the following.

1. **Auditory comprehension of spoken language.** Initially, ask patients to point to named pictures, objects, or body parts. Ask yes/no questions. Later, ask for correct responses to phrases and sentences. Ask them to follow instructions. Gradually, increase the complexity of speech presented to the patients.
2. **Naming responses.** Select names of objects, persons, and actions that are of immediate use to the client. Besides, synonyms and antonyms, rhyming words, spelling selected words, and completing sentences with target words may all be useful targets.
3. **Phrases and sentences.** Initial targets may be useful phrases and simple sentences. Subsequently, expand the repertoire by adding a variety of sentence forms or functional units including mands (requests, commands, demands), tacts or declarative statements, wh-questions, yes-no questions, passives, and other forms. Include specific morphologic features necessary for these verbal expressions.
4. **Pragmatic aspects of language.** Teach such conversational behaviors as turn taking, topic maintenance, and narration as found appropriate.
5. **Gestures paired with verbal expressions.** If it improves communication, pair ordinary gestures or a formal system of gestures (e.g, AMERIND) with words and sentences.
6. **Writing.** Copying letters, words, and sentences; writing from dictation and spontaneous writing are the typical targets often taught in that order.
7. **Reading skills.** First, teach reading isolated words that are useful to the patient. Next, teach silent reading (and comprehension) of materials of high interest and pragmatic value.

Select reading passages from graded materials. Target more complex and longer reading passages as the patient's comprehension of read information improves.

Target Behaviors for Patients With Verbal Apraxia. Verbal apraxia is a motor speech disorder involving difficulty in initiating and executing movement patterns necessary to produce speech even though there is no paralysis, weakness, or discoordination of speech muscles. It is a disorder of both articulation and prosody (Rosenbeck, 1985). The difficulty is thought to be due to impaired motor planning of speech.

Apraxia of speech may be caused by damage to the motor programmer in the brain. Apraxia also may result from edima or damage to tissue surrounding the motor programmer. Apraxia may be associated with aphasia and dysarthrias as well. In such cases, treatment targets include those that are appropriate for aphasic and dysarthric patients as well.

Depending on the pattern of errors and problems of the individual patient, target some or all of the following behaviors for treatment.

1. **Nonspeech movements.** Target these for patients who cannot imitate speech sounds and syllables. Select those movements that are related to speech: tongue protrusion, blowing, biting the lower lip, pressing the two lips together, tongue tip movements, and so forth. These often are appropriate initial targets for patients with severe apraxia. However, generally, do not start with nonspeech movements unless attempts at starting treatment with speech movements have failed.
2. **Misarticulated but correctly imitated speech sounds.** The initial speech sounds to be treated may be those that are imitated or correctly produced with fewer trials.
3. **Sounds that are produced with visible movements of the articulators.** These are also good initial targets.
4. **Singletons and clusters.** Generally, treat them in that order, but consider the pattern of errors of individual patients.
5. **Most frequently occurring sounds.** Treat them first. Target sounds that are used less frequently or rarely for later treatment.
6. **Stressed syllables.** Select these for treatment if your patient's performance on them is better than that on unstressed syllables. This is true of some patients.
7. **Gesturing and writing.** These are targets especially in the case of severely apraxic patients.
8. **Rhythm.** Use it as in the Melodic Intonation Therapy.

9. **Normal prosody.** Teach normal sounding intonation by systematically varying it during sentence production and continuous speech.

Target Behaviors for Patients With Dysarthrias. Dysarthrias are a group of speech disorders that are due to impaired muscular control of the speech mechanism. This impairment, in turn, is due to brain injury or various neurological diseases. Besides muscular control problems, the symptoms include respiratory, phonatory, resonance, articulatory, and prosodic problems. There are different types of dysarthrias though they share many common characteristics. Targets selected for a client depend on the predominant type of dysarthria and the pattern of difficulties.

Some of the commonly targeted behaviors for most dysarthric patients include.

1. **Appropriate posture and tone, and improved strength of muscles.** Relaxation is targeted when there is hypertonia. Induce postural adjustments that facilitate improved speech. Improved strength of the general musculature may be targeted by the physical therapist, but the speech-language pathologist's target is improved tone of muscles involved in speech production.
2. **Improved respiratory management for speech.** Improved muscle strength and appropriate postural adjustments are interrelated with this target. Teach controlled and sustained exhalation that helps produce sustained and louder speech.
3. **Improved phonatory behaviors.** Treat hyperadduction through relaxation training and hypoadduction through increased muscular effort by such means as pushing exercises.
4. **Improved articulatory skills.** Achieve improved intelligibility of speech through articulation training. Targets are syllables and words rather than sounds.
5. **Improved resonance characteristics.** To achieve this target, reduce hypernasality and increase oral resonance.
6. **Improved prosody.** Teach improved rhythm, stress, and intonation of speech. You may have to teach speech rate control as well.
7. **Nonverbal or augmentative means of communication.** For the severely impaired persons who do not benefit from

verbal communication training, teach nonverbal means of communication. For others, teach augmentative means to supplement oral speech.

Neurogenic Communicative Disorders in Children

A major group of children with neurogenic communicative disorders are classified as cerebral palsied. These children will have suffered brain damage in the prenatal and perinatal period. However, brain damage suffered later in childhood may not be classified as cerebral palsy. The speech problems of the neurologically affected children are called developmental dysarthria.

Brain damage in children is different from that in adults mainly because of their still developing neuromuscular system and communicative behaviors. Even so, many common effects are seen in adults and children with neuropathologies. Children with neuropathologies are a diverse group with varied etiology, symptomatology, and subgroup classifications. Target behaviors selected for a child depend on these factors. Therefore, you should select target behaviors after a careful assessment of both the neurophysiological status and communicative behaviors. Neurologically affected children typically need physiotherapy to improve muscle functioning. Some speech-language pathologists with special training in techniques that promote neuromotor development may combine some of those techniques with communication training methods.

Because neuropathologies affect all aspects of speech, treatment targets include the fundamental processes of speech. Communicative behaviors commonly targeted for children with neuropathologies include the following.

1. **Respiratory management for speech.** Teach the client to inhale a sufficient amount of air for speech, then exhale in a controlled manner to sustain phonation and speech, and to maintain a rhythmic pattern of inhalation and exhalation.
2. **Appropriate phonatory behaviors.** Target appropriate loudness, pitch, and voice quality.
3. **Improved resonance with or without surgical or prosthetic treatment.** Reduce hypernasality and nasal emission, and increase oral resonance.

4. **Improved articulation and intelligibility.** Teach specific speech sounds that are difficult for the individual client. Teach visible sounds, correctly imitated sounds, and sounds that are correctly produced in some contexts before other sounds. You also may consider speech muscle training to improve their strength, tone, and range of motion.
5. **Improved prosody.** Target appropriate stress and intonation to reduce monotonous speech.

Target Behaviors for Children With Developmental Apraxia. In some children, a form of articulation disorder is diagnosed as developmental apraxia. Although adults with apraxia of speech show evidence of brain damage, children with a diagnosis of developmental apraxia do not. Therefore this diagnostic category is controversial (Thompson, 1988).

Select the following target behaviors for the client with a diagnosis of developmental apraxia.

1. **Nonspeech movements of oral structures.** These targets should be related to speech movements.
2. **Imitation of speech sounds.** Initial targets should be visible sounds and the trials should be massed. But do not linger on these targets because isolated sound productions are not a problem for the developmentally apraxic person.
3. **Syllables and words in which the articulatory breakdowns occur.** If the breakdowns occur only in phrases and sentences, start treatment at this level. Use words that require back-to-front and front-to-back articulatory placement (e.g., *back/cab*).
4. **Reduced rate of speech.** The target sounds in words and sentences must be produced at a slower rate and with even stress to achieve improved intelligibility.

Target Behaviors for Persons With Hearing Impairment

Hearing impairment varies from a minimal loss to profound deafness. The degree of effect on communication depends on various factors including the age of onset, the type and degree of loss, the quality and the time of initial intervention, and many others. Even mild hearing impairment in infancy is a potential cause of speech and language problems. Severe to profound loss almost always creates significant problems of speech, language, resonance, prosody, and intelligibility.

Complete audiological and otological examinations and a thorough assessment of all aspects of communication are essential before you select target behaviors for your client who is hearing impaired. Compared to the hard of hearing, the deaf require a more intensive as well as extensive treatment program. The deaf need training on all aspects of speech and language production.

What follows is a list of some commonly targeted speech and language behaviors for persons with communicative problems associated with hearing impairment. These target behaviors are part of a carefully developed program of aural rehabilitation whose major components are the use of amplification, auditory training, and working with the family members.

1. **Oral language.** For the infant with hearing impairment, an early, home-based, language stimulation is started first and formal language training is started as soon as practical. Basic vocabulary and morphologic, syntactic, and pragmatic aspects of language are all targets.
2. **Speech production and improved articulation.** For the infant, the period of language stimulation is also the period of speech stimulation. The child constantly hears the speech sounds in syllables and words. Later, formal speech training is started. Teach all misarticulated target sounds; among these, fricatives, affricates, and those that are produced at the back of the mouth are especially important to teach. Also, teach correct productions of distorted vowels.
3. **Improved voice quality.** Children and adults who are deaf need extensive training in improving their voice quality. You may target reduced hypernasality, improved oral resonance, improved nasal resonance on nasal sounds, reduced nasal emission, and overall improved voice quality.
4. **Improved prosody.** With or without the help of biofeedback devices, teach improved rhythm and intonation of speech. Also, teach modified speech rate, smooth flow of words, and appropriate pitch and loudness.
5. **Non-oral means of communication.** For clients who cannot benefit from oral speech-language training, target non-oral means of communication. Some non-oral systems of communication are described in the next section.

Target Behaviors for Nonverbal Persons

Many children and adults with multiple physical and sensory disabilities may not master the skills of oral language needed for social communication. These people are the candidates for nonverbal means of communication.

Nonverbal persons may be candidates for several modes of communication, but most learn some oral speech. Therefore, in many children and adults, the selected nonverbal modes supplement oral speech and language. For this reason, these modes of communication are called **augmentative**. They augment (enhance, expand) oral speech. In persons with severe disabilities, the nonverbal means may be the primary mode of communication.

There are many modes of nonverbal communication. Each has its advantages and limitations. Select the one that suits the client after a careful assessment of his or her physical potential and limitations, communicative needs, cost of the system, and practicality (Musselwhite & St. Louis, 1988; Silverman, 1989).

The two major means of nonverbal communication are **unaided** and **aided**. Unaided means of communication do not require the use of equipment and include gestures, signs, mime, and facial expression. Incidentally, speech is also unaided communication, but our focus here is on nonverbal means. Aided means of communication use graphic or physical symbols and equipment of various sorts including mechanical and electronic devices.

There are several unaided systems of communication. The following are better known and perhaps more frequently used than several other systems.

1. **American Sign Language (ASL).** Considered a separate language with its own rule system, ASL is the most sophisticated and widely used system of nonverbal communication. You may teach this system to deaf persons because they prefer it.
2. **Signed English.** In this system, signs stand for words and morphologic features. The signs parallel the word order of spoken English.
3. **Signed Exact English.** Another set of signs that closely follows the spoken and written forms of English.
4. **Amer-Ind Gestural Code.** This is not a linguistic or sign system; it is also known as American Indian Hand Talk. It has been used by peoples of different Indian tribes to communicate with each other. It has been an excellent means of intercultural communication.

5. **Fingerspelling.** In this system, words are spelled by fingers; letters are represented by various handshapes.

The aided systems are also many. Because some of the aided systems are based on computer technology, new systems are likely to emerge in the near future. You should keep in touch with recent developments and select the one that is most useful and practical for the particular client. Among the aided systems, some use symbols, pictures, and graphic devices whereas others involve electronic devices. The following are among the ones that may be considered.

1. **Object Display.** Teach the client to communicate by pointing to various objects displayed in front. Use real or miniaturized objects.
2. **Pictures, photographs, and line drawings.** Select commercially available packages or prepare them for individual clients.
3. **Traditional Orthography.** English (or any other language) may be represented on a communication board. You may design boards with the letters of the language and some commonly used words and phrases. The display may be electronic.
4. **Blissymbolics.** These are a collection of semi-iconic and abstract symbols printed and pasted on a communication board. Teach individual symbols that single words and combination of symbols to form phrases and sentences. Because the symbols are not language specific, they may be read by speakers of any language.
5. **Rebuses.** In this system, words or parts of words are represented by pictographic drawings. Some of the drawings are combined with letters of the alphabet; others are more like pictures of the objects or persons.
6. **Abstract Symbol Systems.** There are several symbol systems that use abstract, geometric shapes whose meaning is established only by training; examples are Carrier symbols (Premack-type) or Yerkish Lexigrams. The Premack-type symbols are plastic shapes that may be arranged into phrases and sentences. The Yerkish Lexigrams contain nine geometric figures that may be combined to form messages.
7. **Braille and International Morse Code.** These use traditional orthography. Braille contains a set of tactile symbols (raised dots) traditionally used by blind persons. Morse code is a system of dots and dashes. Messages expressed in Morse

code may be printed in English. You may use computerized electronic devices to translate and print Morse code messages.

8. **Speech Generators or Synthesizers.** These are electronic devices that store messages. The speaker can retrieve these messages and display them on small screens or deliver them through built-in speakers. You may use a computer monitor to display messages.

9. **Neuro-assisted devices.** Use these with the most severely disabled individuals who cannot use their hands or feet to point or type messages or activate switches by movement to deliver messages electronically. These devices do not require the speaker to move or act on the switching mechanism to generate messages. The body's electrical signals activate the device and generate messages. Both muscle action potentials and brain waves have been used to activate specially designed electric typewriters, teletypewriters, and computers. Currently, this technology is expensive and of limited use, but improvements may be expected.

Target behaviors described in this chapter should help you get started with most clients. In all cases, remember that the final treatment target is effective communication in natural settings. Throughout the treatment phase, periodically assess your client's status to find out what additional target behaviors must be taught to enhance communication. Follow the logic of moving from simple behaviors to more complex behaviors, from clinically controlled speech to speech controlled by natural events in the client's environment.

7

Treatment in Speech-Language Pathology: Concepts and Methods

I n speech-language pathology, the term treatment includes medical and educational connotations of treating and teaching persons with communicative disorders. Most importantly, the term is used in its basic scientific sense. **Treatment is an agent of change.** To effect change is the main job of clinicians and educators. Any time you teach a new communicative behavior to someone or alter an existing one, you will have changed that person. Therefore, you will have treated that person.

All treatment or teaching methods are means of creating something that did not exist or changing something that did. We create or alter communicative behaviors. In **speech-language pathology, treatment is rearranging communicative relations between speakers and their listeners.** Success in treating communicative disorders depends on how effectively the clinician changes the way certain speakers and their listeners react to each other.

The rearrangement of the listener-speaker relation begins with the new ways in which the speech-language pathologist organizes his or her interaction with the client (Hegde, 1988). The clinician manipulates stimuli and creates new stimuli that might increase the probability of appropriate communicative behaviors. For example, in the case of a child who is language delayed, the clinician may bring and manipulate various objects, toys, pictures, and other stimuli that might set the stage for speech and language. The clinician may model the correct responses, ask the child to imitate those responses, prompt the child to say something, and perform other acts that might lead to a desirable response.

The rearrangement continues when the clinician responds to the child's attempts at communication in ways that are different from what the child has been accustomed to. While the family members may have responded favorably to a nonverbal child's gestures, the clinician may not. Instead, the clinician may proceed quickly to teach words to replace gestures. When the child begins to reliably produce those target words, the clinician will expect the child to produce words instead of gestures. The clinician may reinforce only the word productions. In this manner, the clinician may change the results of the child's communicative attempts. Words produce more favorable results than gestures. Consequently, the child's communicative attempts change for the better.

The final and probably the most important part of rearranging a communicative relation is to change the way family, friends, and others in the life of a client react to the client. In the case of the child who is language delayed, the clinician teaches family members new ways of interacting with the child. These are the ways the clinician will have used to change the communicative behaviors in the child. Family members, teachers, and friends are taught to react the way the clinician reacted. These persons now should react differently to the child's gestures and words. These differential (discriminated) reactions help support and sustain the newly learned communicative behaviors and help eliminate the old, undesirable behaviors.

Basic Methods of Treatment

To treat disorders of communication, you should perform the following tasks.

1. **Evoke communicative behaviors.** Normally, no special procedures are required to evoke speech from speakers. Speech itself is a powerful stimulus. Also, events surrounding us and our internal body states provide additional stimulus to speak. But in case of persons who are communicatively disordered, typical stimuli are ineffective in evoking speech. We need special procedures.

2. **Create nonexistent communicative behaviors.** Many clients who seek treatment do not produce certain desirable communicative behaviors. The task of the clinician is to create those behaviors. For example, a clinician who treats a child who has not acquired language must create verbal behaviors the child did not produce.

3. **Increase existing communicative behaviors.** Many other clients who seek treatment do have certain communicative behaviors in their repertoire, but the behaviors are not produced frequently enough. In such cases, the clinician's task is to increase the frequency of those behaviors. For instance, a stuttering person does speak fluently, but not often enough.

4. **Strengthen and sustain communicative behaviors.** Communicative behaviors created in the clinic or increased to a higher frequency may not be produced in the natural environment. Also, the newly learned behaviors may not last. Therefore, before dismissing clients from treatment, the clinician must use procedures that help strengthen and sustain newly taught behaviors.

5. **Control undesirable behaviors.** Treatment also includes procedures that help decrease certain behaviors. These include undesirable communicative behaviors and such inappropriate behaviors as uncooperative behaviors, nonattending behaviors, crying, and other behaviors that interfere with treatment. In this chapter, we describe procedures to create, evoke, increase, strengthen, and sustain communicative behaviors. In Chapter 8 we describe procedures to decrease undesirable and uncooperative behaviors.

How To Evoke Communicative Behavior

Evoking procedures are special stimulus events needed to have clients in treatment produce speech. The frequently used evoking procedures include instructions, modeling, prompts, and physical stimuli.

Instructions

Instructions describe the skill to be learned. Technically, instructions set up the target behaviors. Therefore, instructions are the starting point of treatment. We often have to tell the young and the old what we want them to learn. Various instructions are used in treating disorders of articulation, language, voice, and fluency

Instructions in Treating Articulation Disorders. In teaching the correct production of speech sounds, give instructions on how to produce them. Describe tongue positions, lip configurations, direction of airflow, mouth opening or closing, and other actions necessary to produce the target sounds. Also, describe the articulatory movements and contacts needed to produce the target sounds. While giving these instructions, model what you describe.

Following is a sample of instructions given in treatment sessions designed to correct certain kinds of articulation disorders.

In correcting an interdental lisp, you may give the following instructions.

1. I want you to say /ʃ/ (sh). While you are saying it, smile so your lips go like this (demonstrate lip retraction). Then, push your tongue toward your front teeth, like this (demonstrate). Let us see if your /ʃ/ (sh) changes for an /s/.
2. Let me hear you say /i/. OK, now make a long /i/ and as you make it, raise the tip of your tongue to blow the air through the teeth.

In teaching the correct production of /l/, you might try the following instructions.

1. Put the tip of your tongue here (demonstrate the correct tongue position for /l/). Now say /a/ as you lower the tip of your tongue. Did you hear [la]? Good. Repeat that for me.
2. Look at the mirror. Open your mouth like this (demonstrate a slight mouth opening to show the tongue placement). Now say /l/.

In teaching the correct production of /f/, the following instruction may be useful.

1. Bite gently on your lower lip like this (demonstrate). Now as you do it, blow air like this (demonstrate).

Many other kinds of instructions are used in teaching the correct production of various speech sounds. When you select target sounds for a client, give some thought to how you might give instructions to produce them.

Instructions in Treating Language Disorders. Various aspects of language may be treatment targets for children with language delay or disorder, adults with aphasia, and children and adults with inappropriate language. In treating language disorders, instructions may be given about when to use the selected target language feature or element.

Children who have not learned language in the normal process do not begin to produce elements of language when instructed about the rules of usage. For example, a child who does not produce the plural morpheme correctly will not produce it because the clinician has described the rules of plural usage. However, simplified descriptions of certain rules may be helpful when combined with other treatment procedures.

Different kinds of instructions may be equally effective in teaching various elements of language. Therefore, the following examples are only suggestive. You may experiment with other kinds of instructions for the same target behaviors:

Instructions to train the irregular plural morpheme.

When you see one of these (show a picture), you say "Woman." (Say "woman." Good). But when you see two like these, (show a different picture), you say "Women." (Say "women." Good.)

Instructions to train the regular plural morphemes /s/.

When you see one of these (show a picture), you say "cup." (Say "cup." Good.) But when you see two of these (show a different picture), you say "cups." (Say "cups." Good).

Instructions to teach appropriate greeting responses.

Look at the picture here. They are eating breakfast. When it is breakfast time, you say "Good morning." (Say "good morning." Good.) And look at this picture here. They are going to bed. When it is time to sleep, you say "Good night." (Say "Good night." Excellent.)

Instructions to teach correct recall of names to an aphasic person.

When I show this picture (the client's daughter) and ask you who is this, say "Nina." (Say "Nina." Very good.) But when I show this picture (the client's son), and ask who is this, say "Tom." (Say "Tom." That was correct!)

In preparing instructions for a client in language treatment, do not describe grammatic rules in linguistic terms though you will be teaching behaviors that may seem to follow such rules. It is not helpful for a client to hear you say that "Gerunds are special forms of verbs that end in *ing*." The clients (and all speakers of any language) do not have to know the linguistic name of a grammatic feature to use it correctly.

In some cases, you may describe the conditions under which a feature is used. For example, instead of describing the rules of verb usage, you may demonstrate actions and describe them to show when certain verbs are used. Whenever possible, make the conditions of usage concrete; use pictures and arranged situations; when you instruct rules of conversations, engage in conversations to exemplify them.

Instructions in Treating Voice Disorders. Treatment of voice disorders in adults and children requires many instructions. Mostly, treatment targets in voice therapy include changes in vocal quality, pitch, loudness, or resonance. In all cases, first you must instruct your clients about the particular target and how to achieve it. Once the target behavior is established in the clinic, you need to implement additional procedures to document its reliable occurrence in the natural environment and to sustain it over time. These procedures, too, require the use of instructions.

In treating clients with vocal hyperfunction, sometimes changing the head position while talking may be beneficial. In such cases, you might give instructions of the following kind.

> The position of your head while talking affects your voice. A change in head position may improve your voice. Let us try. (Experiment with different head positions while the client produces prolonged vowels to see if a desirable change occurs.) Now it sounds like your voice improves when you flex your neck downward so that your chin almost touches your chest. Keep your head in that position and say /i/. Does your voice sound better? Good.

In treating clients with reduced oral resonance, talking with a greater mouth opening is often recommended. In this case, explanation and instruction of the following kind may be used.

> When you talk with closed mouth, your voice sounds muffled. It sounds better if you keep your mouth open while talking. Let us try. Say /a/ while you open your mouth widely. Drop your jaw and make the sound. Now close your jaw and make the same sound. Do you hear a difference? Good. Let us now practice making sounds and saying words while keeping the mouth open.

To reduce a child's vocally abusive behaviors, first you have to establish the frequency of those behaviors. For example, a child may spend much time playing with toy guns. While playing, he or she may also produce tensed and loud phonation. **To establish the frequency of this vocally abusive behavior, you may instruct the parent as follows.**

> During the next week, I would like you to chart how often your son (or daughter) plays with the toy guns making the loud sounds you have described to me. Also, chart how long he (or she) played each time. Record the date and the beginning and ending time of each episode. Once we know how often he (or she) engages in this behavior, we can design a plan to reduce it.

An adult man who has been treated to **talk with a lower pitch** in the clinic may be asked to document its maintenance in the natural environment. In this case, you may instruct the client as follows.

> I would like you to keep a record of how often you used your new pitch. Anytime you talked in your old pitch, make a note on this card (give the client a recording sheet or card). Also, anytime you lower the pitch, make a note. Make this kind of record for a week and bring it to the next session.

In preparing instruction for clients with voice disorders, first select the target vocal behavior and find out how that behavior may be facilitated. Make sure the selected facilitating technique works; experiment informally. Find out more about this approach in the section on **Shaping Voice Characteristics** (see p.177–178).

Instructions in Treating Fluency Disorders. In treating disorders of fluency, including stuttering and cluttering, instructions and demonstrations play a major role. In most stuttering treatment programs, you need to teach skills of fluent speech production. As described in Chapter 6, the most frequently used target behaviors include management of airflow, gentle phonatory onset, and reduced rate of speech through syllable stretching.

In teaching appropriate airflow management, give the following instructions.

> I would like you to breathe in a bit more air than the usual. Like this. (Demonstrate a deeper than the usual inhalation.) Then, immediately let a little bit of air through your mouth. Like this. (Demonstrate a slight exhalation through open mouth.) You try it. Make sure you do not hold the air in your lungs. As soon as you breathe in, breathe out a small amount of air.

In teaching gentle phonatory onset, you may instruct the client as follows.

> Sometimes you start your sound abruptly and harshly. Your vocal cords work too hard when you do this. You experience too much muscular tension and effort when you start sounds abruptly and harshly. Instead, you should start your sound softly, easily, and with less effort and tension. Let us practice that.

In teaching rate reduction through syllable stretching, use the following instructions.

> You may have noticed that when you speak slowly, your fluency improves. Practicing a slower rate of speech is part of our treatment program. You do not want to slow down your speech by pausing between words. (Demonstrate this.) Instead, I would like you to reduce your overall rate by stretching the syllables of words. I want you to stretch most syllables, but the first syllable of the first few words in a sentence must be stretched more than the other syllables. Like this. (Demonstrate syllable stretching.)

A reduced rate also improves the fluency and intelligibility of a speaker with cluttering. In general, stuttering treatment procedures may be modified in treating cluttering.

How To Prepare Effective Instructions

The client understands the target behaviors only by your instructions and demonstrations. Unless you give effective instructions, the rest of the treatment procedures may be difficult to implement. Therefore, use the following general guidelines in preparing and delivering your instructions.

1. Select the target behavior.
2. Make an analysis of the target behavior. What topographic features distinguish the behavior? In other words, what is the shape or the form of the target behavior? How does it look, feel, or sound?
3. Find out how the target behavior can be evoked. Generally, simplify it so it can be produced by the client.
4. Write out instructions that help evoke the target behavior. Write them in simple, clear, and unambiguous words; whenever possible, use ordinary language. Especially for children, write instructions in words they can understand.
5. Do not talk down to the client. Modify your presentation depending on the judged level of the client's sophistication.

6. Rehearse the instructions. Once you gain experience, you can give instructions spontaneously. In the beginning of your clinical practicum, you should practice giving instructions before you give them to your client.

7. Do not read instructions to your client; do not deliver instructions too formally. Deliver instructions in a natural, conversational manner.

8. Make sure the client understands your instructions. Ask the the client to repeat your instructions. See if the client can do what you ask him or her to do. If not, repeat your instructions, change words, add gestures, and demonstrate.

9. Repeat all or portions of your instructions whenever the client makes mistakes that suggest that the instructions are not remembered.

10. Give new instructions whenever you change the target behavior or you shift training to a higher level.

Modeling

Modeling, like instructions and other stimulus events, is a necessary part of treatment in communicative disorders. When the client does not respond correctly with instructions and other stimuli, you have to model the target response. Clinical research has shown that modeling is an effective procedure in establishing many kinds of target behaviors. Therefore, modeling is one of the widely used methods of teaching new behaviors.

In some language treatment programs, the clinician may model target responses, but may not necessarily expect the child to imitate it. In most other treatment sessions, the clinician expects the client to imitate the modeled response. Note that modeling is the special stimulus provided by the clinician and imitation is the response given to this stimulus. Because imitation is a client's response, it never should be described as a treatment procedure. Modeling is a treatment procedure because it is provided by the clinician to evoke the imitated response.

Normally, a stimulus and its response are topographically different. For example, the stimulus "How are you doing?" is topographically different from the response "Fine, thank you." To be called imitation, a response should meet two criteria. First, **imitated response should be topographically similar to the modeled stimulus**. Ideally, the stimulus and the response should be identical. But in clinical training, modeling and imitation may not be identical, especially in the beginning stage. Yet, an acceptable imitation and its stimulus (modeling) should have a similar form. In case of vocal and verbal behaviors, the two should sound similar. If not, there is no imitation.

Second, imitated response should follow the modeled stimulus immediately. Though delayed imitation sometimes is described in the literature, the most clinically useful imitation is immediate. This is because the clinician can reinforce the immediately imitated response. Obviously, the clinician cannot reinforce the client who repeats the modeled response at another time and place. Possibly, no individual may reinforce that response.

Modeling in the Treatment of Communicative Disorders. Probably, modeling is most frequently used in the treatment of **articulation disorders**. When the sounds are taught in words or in isolation, modeling is most useful. Before modeling the target sound, you may instruct the client on how to produce it. While giving such instructions, you will have modeled the correct production of the target sound. After giving instructions and demonstrations, ask the client to imitate the sound you modeled. You may also consider playing taped models for the client to imitate. Taped models provide standard stimuli; a collection of such stimuli may be useful in treating articulation disorders.

In treating **language disorders**, modeling is better preceded by the question which alone should eventually evoke the response. For example, in teaching the regular plural morpheme with the help of pictures, you should not just show the picture of two books and model "*books*" for the client to imitate. You should ask a question and then model the correct response. In the same example, you should ask a question such as "*What do you see?*" or "*What are these?*" and immediately model the response by saying "*Say books.*" Similarly, in teaching words to children who are language delayed, you should show a picture or an object, ask a question, and immediately model the response. For example: "*What is this? Say cat.*"

When a question reliably precedes modeling, the correct response may be maintained later when modeling is withdrawn and only the question is asked. For example, assume the child consistently imitates "*books,*" when you say "*What are these? Say books.*" Then, you stop modeling and ask "*What are these?*" The child may say "*books.*" If you did not ask the question before modeling the response, the question, introduced later, may not evoke the correct response because it is a new stimulus to which the child previously has not responded.

When the client imitates the target response consistently, you should stop modeling. Yet, when the modeled stimulus suddenly is stopped, even after the client has been imitating the target response, the response may not be produced. This is likely to happen especially when the modeled target responses are long, as they often are when the targets are grammatic features. Therefore, in many cases, you should **fade the modeled stimulus**.

In fading a modeled stimulus, withdraw parts of it. Withdraw additional parts as the correct response is maintained. For example, in teaching the preposition on, you may have asked the question "Where is the ball?" and modeled *"Say the ball is on the table."* Note that the modeled stimulus is a long sentence that included other syntactic elements. In fading this modeled stimulus, first you should drop the last word. After asking the question, you model *"Say the ball is on the . . . ,"* and wait for the correct response. Ask the child to start with *"The ball"* as the likely response is just *"table."* If the child gives the correct response (the entire sentence), then on the next trial, drop another word by modeling only *"Say the ball is on. . . ."* Make sure the child repeats the whole target sentence. On each of the subsequent trials, drop one additional word of the modeled phrase until you ask only the question *"Where is the ball?"*

Treatment of **voice disorders** also requires extensive modeling. The desired pitch, loudness, vocal quality, and resonance characteristics must be modeled for the client. In some cases, the clinician may be unable to model a desired voice characteristic. For example, an adult male may not be able to model a target vocal pitch for a child or a woman. In such cases, the model voice may be tape recorded from another child or woman and played for the client to imitate. Also, clients themselves may provide voice models. A patient with too high a pitch may be able to produce a lower pitch with some help from the clinician. This desired pitch may be tape recorded and used as a model for the client to imitate. With appropriate software and such instruments as Visi-Pitch, many voice characteristics may be displayed on computer monitors.

In treating **stuttering and cluttering**, varied behaviors are targeted. In teaching such fluency skills as management of airflow, reduced rate of speech, and gentle phonatory onset, you should first model each skill separately and then in combination. For example, you may start with inhalation and a slight exhalation before saying a word or two. Therefore, model as you describe inhalation and exhalation. You then add rate reduction by describing and modeling it. Thus, you put together all the components of treatment targets.

How To Model Effectively

A clear model, produced by the clinician or a mechanical device, can be effective in treatment. With some clients, repeated modeling is indispensable. Use the following guidelines in providing effective modeling and to determine when to model, how much to model, and when to stop modeling.

1. Decide whether you will model the target response or whether taped or otherwise mechanically represented model will be used. Possibly, as clinical instrumentation becomes more sophisticated and more commonly used, mechanical models will be used more frequently. If your clinic has such instruments, use mechanical models.

2. If a client's own correct response can serve as a model, use it.

3. Model often in the early stages of treatment because it is needed to establish the target behavior.

4. Model consistently and continuously in the beginning until the imitated responses are produced reliably. Use such objective criteria as *production of five consecutively correct imitated responses* before terminating modeling. Do not terminate modeling prematurely; this will unnecessarily increase the error rate.

5. Do not overuse modeling. Do not continue modeling when the client meets an objective criterion (such as five correctly imitated responses). Remember that the final target is not imitated responses but responses given to more natural stimuli.

6. Reinstate modeling when the client fails to give the correct response without it. Do not continue to evoke wrong responses by not providing the needed modeling. Reinstate modeling when two to four wrong responses are given on trials without modeling.

7. Instead of stopping suddenly, fade the complex and lengthy model. If the wrong responses return the instant you stop modeling, then drop the final element first and work your way backwards until all elements of the modeled stimulus are faded and only the question is asked.

8. Model every new target response when first introduced.

9. Model the same target response when training is moved to a higher level. For example, model the /s/ in words when you shift training from syllable to word level. Model the phoneme in phrases, and again in sentences when the training is shifted to these higher levels.

10. Reduce the frequency of modeling in the final stages of treatment. Use it least frequently when the target response is stabilized in conversational speech.
11. Ask the client to imitate your model promptly.
12. Reinforce the imitated responses. In the beginning, reinforce approximations of the model, but reinforce only promptly produced responses. On subsequent trials, reinforce progressively better approximations until the response matches the model.

Prompting

Prompts and models are similar in one important respect. Both are special stimuli that precede the target response. In all other respects, models and prompts are different.

A prompt is often a partial stimulus whereas a modeled stimulus is full-fledged. For example, when you model, you might say "Jimmy, say *the cat is jumping*"; but when you prompt the same response, you might say "Jimmy, *the cat is* . . . ." and wait for the response. All models are direct stimuli; they display the full response. **Some prompts are indirect stimuli**; they only suggest the target response instead of displaying it. For instance, to model a slower rate of speech for a stutterer, you have to speak slowly to fully display it. But to prompt it, you may raise your finger to signal a slower rate. Some prompts may contain parts of the target response while others may contain no part of it. For instance, your prompt "Jimmy, the cat is. . . ," contains some parts of the target response. But a hand gesture to slow down the rate of speech contains no part of the target response.

Prompts are imitated to the extent they contain the target response. Many prompts are never imitated because they do not contain the target response at all. When you give a hand gesture to lower the pitch of the voice, for example, the client does not imitate your hand gesture. The client lowers the pitch of his or her voice. Finally, **some prompts are a special feature of modeled responses**. For example, you might place an extra vocal emphasis on the target preposition *on* when you model "Say the ball is on the table." This vocal emphasis is a prompt within a modeled stimulus.

Besides vocal emphasis, there are many other prompts that help trigger a target response that may be slow in coming. Also, vocal emphasis can take many forms. Vocal emphasis highlights a target response to make it stand out in some way. For example, when a particular target, such as a grammatic feature, is a part of a long string of words, you can highlight the specific target by slightly increasing your vocal intensity on it. In the sentence "Say *the ball is on the table,*" the word *on* would sound slightly louder than the rest of the words. Another method of making the target word distinct is to say it more slowly than the rest of the words. Yet another method of emphasis is to pause briefly just before the production of the target response. Finally, you can say the target response with a slightly different pitch. You can invent other ways of making the target feature stand out from the rest of the modeled response.

Verbal prompts that do not include the target response may be effective when the response has been learned to a certain extent. For example, you may have taught a nonverbal child to name a few pictures. The child may name pictures correctly on some trials but not on other trials. When the child does not respond to your question, you may ask an additional prompting question. Such questions as *"What is the name of this?"* or *"Do you remember what we called this?"* may prompt the correct response. Such verbal clues like *"this word starts with an es"* also may prompt a response.

Several other kinds of prompts are nonverbal. Gestures and motor behaviors, while suggesting the target response, can prompt responses. When you teach verbs, you can demonstrate action to prompt the correct word response. For example, the word *jump* may be prompted by a hopping motion demonstrated by your hand. You may prompt the correct production of a phoneme by showing the correct articulatory posture without saying the sound or the word. For example, you can prompt the correct production of /m/ in *"Mommy"* by pressing the two lips together.

In treating voice disorders, various hand gestures may prompt higher or lower pitch, increased or decreased vocal intensity, presence or absence of nasal resonance, reduced rate of speech, and many other targets.

Prompts should be strong enough to evoke the response but not unnecessarily strong, loud, or long. A prompt is a gentle hint. It is a minimal clue sufficient to evoke a response. Most clients find subtle prompts more acceptable than boisterous prompts. If a brief and quiet hand gesture can prompt a lower rate of speech in a stutterer, avoid lengthy verbal prompts or exaggerated nonverbal prompts.

Teaching clients to respond to subtle prompts is important to later promote maintenance of target responses. As clients learn to produce target behaviors in the clinic, you need to train family members, friends, teachers, and others to evoke those behaviors at home, school, and other places. Clients are likely to find loud and lengthy prompts in these natural settings unpleasant or embarrassing because such clues are obvious to other persons. When family members and others give unobtrusive clues, clients are more likely to respond. If such prompts have been established already by the clinician, the job of family members and others is much easier.

Like modeling, prompts also should be faded. When you observe a few consecutively correct responses to prompts, stop prompting to see if the responses will be maintained. If not, reinstate prompts. Fade prompts by reducing their topography. For example, make a particular hand gesture progressively smaller until it is completely faded out. A lengthy verbal prompt (e.g., *"What do you say for this?"*) may be reduced by using only some of the words or by word substitutions (e.g., *"You say . . ."* or *"This is . . ."*).

How To Prompt Effectively

Prompting at the right time with the right clue will reduce the frequency of wrong responses. Use the following guidelines in using this technique effectively.

1. Whenever appropriate, use partial modeling to prompt the target responses. This will help fade modeling and keep the correct response rate high.
2. Give your prompts promptly. Delayed prompts may promote delayed responses. The earliest sign of a hesitation or a wrong response is your clue to prompt.
3. Prompt more frequently in the beginning stages of treatment. Gradually reduce its frequency as the correct responses become more stable and the responding becomes faster.
4. Prefer a subtle or short prompt over a loud or lengthy prompt. Prefer a silent, gestural prompt over a verbal prompt.
5. Fade prompts by making them progressively subtler or shorter.
6. Teach family members to prompt the target behaviors in a subtle manner.

Physical Stimuli

Instructions, modeling, and prompts can help evoke target behaviors in most clients. But some clients need additional stimuli. Children and adults in language therapy often need physical stimuli. In teaching words and various elements of grammar, pictures or objects may be necessary to evoke target responses. Physical stimuli may be helpful in articulation treatment as well.

The clients who are developmentally disabled, nonverbal, or multiply handicapped may need physical stimuli the most. In some cases, the selection of initial target responses may depend on whether they can be depicted concretely. In the beginning stages of treatment, elements of language that can be represented through pictures or objects are taught more easily than those that are abstract. Words that name everyday objects and events also are useful targets to such clients.

Pictures and objects may be used to evoke speech from children in treatment sessions. In the final stages of treatment, the clinician must evoke continuous speech from all clients. Target behaviors must be stabilized in conversational speech to promote maintenance. Children who are reluctant to talk may begin to talk when you show them pictures in story books.

Though pictures and objects are useful stimuli, you should avoid a few mistakes made by some clinicians in using them. A common mistake is to overuse pictures. Some clinicians just cannot talk to their young clients unless they have picture cards to show. Even in the final stages of treatment, when they should carry on a conversation with their clients, clinicians may show pictures and evoke only limited responses. Another mistake is to use poorly drawn commercial pictures instead of taking colorful, realistic pictures from magazines. Pictures in magazine advertisements are more attractive to children than gray shades of line drawings. Yet another mistake is to use pictures when real objects can be used just as easily. Especially in teaching basic words to children, objects are immediately meaningful and direct.

When objects are used as stimuli, the child is more likely to produce the newly learned words at home where the same or similar objects may be encountered. Therefore, objects may promote an initial generalization and subsequent maintenance of newly learned communicative behaviors. The maintenance potential of objects may be enhanced further if the child were to bring objects from his or her own home. The clinician can then use them as stimuli for target responses. In this case, the child takes home the therapeutic stimuli.

How To Effectively Use Physical Stimuli

Most adult clients with conversational skills do not need physical stimuli to evoke target responses or to maintain continuous speech. When concrete representation of target responses is needed, physical stimuli are unavoidable. Therefore, use the following guidelines in the selection and use of physical stimuli.

1. Prefer objects over pictures. If at all practical, ask the child to bring the relevant stimulus objects from home.
2. Select pictures that are three-dimensional, colorful, and realistic.
3. Use pictures and objects in the early stages of treatment. In later stages, especially when continuous speech is evoked, do not use pictures or use them sparingly. When the child is capable of continuous speech, do not use pictures. Find other ways of making the child talk. Talk about what interests the child.
4. If you need to use pictures in story books, read the story to the child and ask him or her to retell the story while looking at the pictures.
5. Discontinue the use of pictures as soon as possible.

Creating New Responses

Many clients with severe physical disabilities resulting in communicative impairments cannot imitate modeled responses. Due to neurological problems, clients may be unable to move their articulators. Children who are nonverbal also are unable to imitate verbal responses. In treating such clients, you cannot just model the target response and expect them to imitate it. A response that is not even imitated is nonexistent in the client's repertoire. You need procedures to create new responses that do not exist.

Shaping or **successive approximation** is a highly researched method of creating new responses. The method allows you to shape a nonexistent complex response from simple responses that do exist in the client's repertoire. In each of several successive stages of treatment, you teach a simple response that takes the client one step closer to the final target response.

Breaking a target response into its simpler components is the key to shaping it. Even the most severely involved client may be able to make some movement that is remotely related to the target response. You then start with this movement and shape something more complex out of it by adding other components. The basic idea in shaping is that you teach what the client can learn in each step. But they are not random responses that the client happens to learn. You teach responses that are systematically related to the final target behavior. Each new response mastered by the client should be a movement in the right direction.

Shaping is not a single, unitary procedure. Being a collection of procedures, it includes differential reinforcement of correct responses, withholding reinforcement for an earlier component while a subsequent component is being taught, and manual guidance. Reinforcement procedures are described later in the chapter.

Manual guidance is physical assistance in shaping a response. When the client cannot make a physical movement at all, you may have to manually assist that movement and reinforce the client for any success. In manual guidance, you gently but firmly make a movement happen. For example, a boy with a severe articulation disorder may not move his tongue tip for an articulatory position. But the movement is possible, only it is not probable. Therefore, you may take a tongue depressor and move the tongue tip in the desired direction. A woman with aphasia may have great difficulty in moving her hand to point to a message on an electronic display, but the movement can be assisted by taking her hand and pointing to the message. When a boy who is profoundly retarded does not open his mouth to produce a vowel, you apply a downward pressure on the chin to make the jaw drop so the mouth is opened. A man with a high-pitched voice does not produce or imitate voice of lower pitch, but as you apply a slight finger pressure on the thyroid cartilage when he produces a prolonged vowel, his pitch may drop. These are all techniques of manual guidance that help shape a target response.

Shaping Correct Articulation Shaping may be necessary in treating many children with severe articulation problems. To shape target phonemes, analyze them to identify their simpler components. Then, find out if the client can perform any of the components that may be used to shape the target phoneme. For example, if your client, a boy with a severe articulation problem, cannot produce a phoneme in words, can he produce it in syllables? If not in syllables, can he produce it in isolation? If not in isolation, can he move the tongue tip in the right direction? Can he make an appropriate lip movement? Can he make any kind of movement of the articulators? Can he open his mouth? If not, can you make him open his mouth with manual guidance? Can you make his tongue or lips move with manual guidance?

As you can see, in shaping, you think of a target behavior as a collection of responses, some of which are more complex than others. The first task is to find one of these responses that the client can perform. If a more complex response cannot be performed, find the next simpler response. If that, too, cannot be performed, simplify the response further until the client can perform a component of the target behavior with or without manual guidance.

After the correct movement of the articulators is achieved, the acoustic properties of the response must be added. For example, when the tongue tip is in the right position, you may ask the client to blow air to produce /s/. In producing voiced sounds, vocalization must be added. A speech sound not produced may be shaped from some kind of sound the child can produce. For example, in shaping /s/ from /ʃ/ (sh), you ask the child to produce the /ʃ/ (sh) and then push the tongue forward until an /s/ is heard.

Shaping Language Behaviors. Children who are nonverbal and those with severe movement problems are excellent candidates for shaping. Simple, single word utterances are the most likely initial targets for these clients. When a certain number of such words are taught, you can combine them into phrases and sentences. The most difficult part of treatment will be this initial stage of establishing a set of basic words. The need for shaping is greatest in this stage.

In teaching word productions to children who are nonverbal who do not imitate words or syllables, first you should find an articulatory movement that can be made. For example, a girl who is nonverbal may be able to open her mouth with manual guidance. With some gentle, downward pressure exerted on her chin, you may get her to open her mouth. Next, as the mouth opens, you may ask her to expel some air through the mouth. Model this, and give some manual assistance; a slight push on the abdomen as the mouth opens will result in some audible expulsion of air. This audible airflow may be a basis to shape an /h/. In the successive stages, you can shape the articulatory movement for /l/ and /o/. You gradually can shape these responses into a *Hello*.

Each target word must be analyzed for simpler components that can be taught. Each component learned should be one step taken in the direction of achieving the final target response. In most cases, start with modeling a basic articulatory posture; give manual guidance if necessary; reinforce the imitated response even if it is only an approximation of the model given; then model the next response; and reinforce the client for correct imitation.

When the client learns a few single words, teach two-word phrases. The same modeling, imitation, and differential reinforcement procedures are used. The client should not need manual guidance at this stage as the individual words are mastered. In subsequent stages, shape first shorter and then longer sentences by adding morphological and syntactic features.

Shaping Voice Characteristics. Many clients with voice disorders may be unable to produce or imitate target voice characteristics. To induce changes in pitch, loudness, resonance, and voice quality, clinicians typically use shaping. Clinicians also use manual guidance which is often described as digital manipulation in textbooks on voice disorders (Boone & McFarlane, 1988).

As mentioned earlier, applying a slight finger pressure on the thyroid cartilage as the client produces a prolonged vowel tends to lower the pitch. The lower pitch is a result of increased mass of vocal folds due to their shortening as the digital pressure pushes the thyroid in the backward direction. Once the client achieves a lower pitch on a vowel, you must shape the pitch in producing words and phrases. The new pitch must be practiced in successively longer utterances until it is sustained in conversational speech.

In experimenting with different head positions that might facilitate a more normal sounding voice, manual guidance may be necessary. You might manually help the client change the head position to change a certain characteristic of voice. Keeping the head straight, tilting it toward left or right side, or flexing the neck in a downward direction are all useful in changing vocal characteristics. In some cases, along with instructions and modeling, manual guidance also may be necessary.

Shaping is a primary technique of voice therapy. In effecting changes in fundamental frequency (pitch), vocal intensity (loudness), oral or nasal resonance, hard glottal attacks, hoarseness, and harshness, you may have to use shaping in the initial stages of treatment. A male speaker's high pitch is reduced in small steps. Any reduction in pitch is reinforced initially. In subsequent steps, speaking with progressively lower pitch is reinforced. The process is continued until the most desirable pitch is established. In most cases, the first step might be to produce a slightly lower pitch on single words. In the next step, the new or even lower pitch is practiced while speaking short phrases. Finally, the lower pitch is used in sentences and conversational speech. A sequence similar to this may be effective in shaping other voice targets.

In shaping target voice characteristics, you might use mechanical devices that give automatic feedback to the client. For example, Visi-Pitch, PM 100 Pitch Analyzer, and Phonatory Function Analyzer may be used in modifying the pitch of a client. An instrument called Tonar II may be used to modify nasal resonance (Boone & McFarlane, 1988). These devices work on the principle of shaping. In each successive step of treatment, the client achieves a progressively higher or lower pitch, decreased or increased nasal resonance, and so forth.

Shaping Fluency. In treating stuttering and cluttering, skills of fluent speech are shaped in sequenced steps. Whether it is management of airflow, gentle phonatory onset, or reduced rate of speech, you must take one skill at a time and shape it. Then you put them together and have the client practice the skills starting at the one- or two-word level. As the client maintains fluency, more complex responses are introduced until fluent speech is practiced in conversational speech outside the clinic. This sequence of treatment also is based on shaping.

To reduce stuttering, you must teach interrelated skills. Therefore, shaping is important. In the beginning, you may start with inhalation and slight exhalation before phonatory onset. This skill may be practiced without phonation. Then, add gentle phonatory onset. Ask the client to produce a syllable or a word. When the airflow management and gentle onset are established, add rate reduction by syllable stretching. Single words are targets at this stage. Before saying the word, the client inhales, exhales slightly, achieves smooth onset, and speaks by stretching the syllables. The initial syllables and vowels must be especially stretched.

When single-word utterances are free from stuttering, ask the client to produce two-word phrases. Monitor all the skills taught so far. If the client maintains speech free from stuttering, have the client practice skills of fluent speech while producing sentences and conversational speech.

An important part of most stuttering treatment programs is to shape normal sounding prosody when stutter-free speech is established. Rate reduction through syllable stretching induces a monotonous speech which is unacceptable in the natural environment. The client is unlikely to speak at that slow rate outside the clinic. This means that fluency may not be maintained. To strengthen fluency at near-normal rate of speech, you should fade the excessively slow rate and shape normal prosody.

By allowing the client to slightly increase the rate, you can make sure that fluency is maintained while shaping normal prosody. In carefully planned steps, allow the rate to increase. Typically, increased rate brings back normal patterns of intonation. In some cases, you may have to shape intonation as well. Shaping pitch variations in conversational speech will be usually effective. Excessively slow speech tends to be too soft. Therefore, shaping louder speech will also help in reducing monotone.

How To Effectively Use Shaping

As you have seen, carefully planned steps in which progressively more complex communicative behaviors are shaped are essential in the treatment of speech, language, voice, and fluency problems. Therefore, use the following general guidelines is shaping target communicative behaviors.

1. Select the final target behavior for the client. Make an analysis of this behavior so you know how to simplify it. Remember that the simplification of a target behavior is client-specific. That is, the same target phoneme, language feature, voice characteristic, or skill of fluency will have to be simplified more or less and in different ways to suit the individual client. But you should know the several ways of simplifying target communicative behaviors.

2. Experiment with the client to find out what relevant response the client can imitate. This will be the initial response to be taught. If a more complex response related to the final target can be imitated, do not select a simpler response. Simplify a response only to the extent needed, not to the extent possible. This is because you have to move the client through the simpler to the more complex final response. Generally, the more complex the initial level, the faster the treatment progress.

3. Teach progressively more complex responses; but always make sure the client is moving in the direction of the final target response.

4. Use instructions, modeling, and manual guidance at each step of training.

5. Reinforce imitated responses. To begin with, accept approximations of modeled responses. Subsequently, reinforce more accurate productions. Do not reinforce the initial and intermediate responses excessively. If you do, you will have difficulty moving the client to higher levels of training. Stabilize only the final target response.

6. Fade modeling and instructions. Also, fade any undesirable aspects of the shaped response. For example, fade the slow rate and the monotone of the treated stutterer. Fade any unusual postures you may have taught to sustain a certain voice quality.

Increasing the Frequency of Responses

Instructions, modeling, and shaping are useful in creating nonexistent communicative behaviors. But these procedures will not be effective if the client's responses do not meet certain consequences. A response may be imitated or produced otherwise. It may be a crude approximation of the modeled response, a perfectly imitated response, or a correct, unimitated response. In each case, the response may not last if certain environmental consequences do not follow it.

How to make certain consequences follow a response is the topic of this section. These consequences help increase the frequency of newly established responses. The consequences also help strengthen and sustain responses taught in treatment sessions. In this section, you will learn about procedures to increase the frequency of new responses. In the next section, you will learn about procedures to strengthen and sustain responses.

Positive Reinforcement

Normally, what the listener does when a speaker says something is the consequence for the speaker's speech. One person (a speaker) may say "Hi!" and the other (listener) may either say "Hi!" or ignore the speaker. The child might say "Mommy!" and the mother may pick up the child. Therefore, in everyday conversations, one person's speech is followed by another person's speech or nonspeech behavior. These behaviors are the consequences of speech. And, these consequences will determine whether the speaker will say the same thing next time.

In treatment, especially in the initial stages, the communicative behaviors and what follow them are not as naturalistic as they typically are. For one thing, the communicative behaviors may be either absent or not effective; that is why the client is seeking help from the clinician. A child who is nonverbal, a woman with aphasia, a man with laryngectomy, and a person who stutters need to do something different in their attempts at communication. Therefore, clinicians set up target behaviors for them. Normally, you only respond to a speaker's communicative behavior. But clinically, you also teach them what or how to say and then you react to it in ways that are "clinical." These clinical ways of reacting to client's speech or attempts at speech are the consequences that either increase or decrease the client's speaking behavior.

There are two kinds of consequences. One kind, when it follows a response, makes the response more likely under similar circumstances. The other kind makes the response less likely in the future. These consequences help decrease undesirable behaviors and are described in chapter 8.

Those consequences that follow a response and increase its frequency are called **positive reinforcers**. The **procedure** of increasing responses by making positive reinforcers follow them is called **positive reinforcement**. To increase the frequency of new target responses, you must reinforce them positively.

In using the positive reinforcement procedure, you must be clear about two factors. First, you should know the correct definition of the procedure and of reinforcers. There are many events that are known to increase the frequency of responses. But none will do it at all times and with all clients. Therefore, initially, select a **potential reinforcer**, arrange it as a consequence for a response, and watch what happens. Count the number of responses produced by the client when the consequence is being used. If the response rate increases, then you call that consequence a reinforcer. If the response rate did not increase, your potential reinforcer was not a reinforcer for that client on that occasion. Note that reinforcers always are defined after they are demonstrated to increase a response rate. Nothing is a reinforcer before such demonstration. Therefore, call an event a reinforcer only after it has increased a rate of response.

Second, you should know that a reinforcer should follow a response immediately. Delayed response consequences do not reinforce as well as immediate consequences. Therefore, recognize the correct response quickly and reinforce promptly.

There are many types of potential positive reinforcers. All are known to be effective some of the time with some clients under certain conditions. You will have to find out whether any of them will work with your clients. You probably will find what the research has shown. Most of them will work with clients on certain occasions. What worked with a client during one treatment session may not work in another session. What worked with one client may not work with another client. Some of the consequences are more powerful than others. No consequence will work with everyone every time.

Primary Reinforcers. Events that increase a response rate because of their biological (survival) value are called primary reinforcers. Potential primary reinforcers include food and escape from or avoidance of unpleasant and injurious situations.

Primary reinforcers that have their effect through escape or avoidance are called **negative reinforcers**. When you run away from a thief in the alley, you escape from an unpleasant (or much worse) experience. Your running behavior will have been reinforced because running helped you escape from an aversive experience. Next time, you probably will run sooner and faster. Better yet, you may totally avoid alleys. This avoidance also will be negatively reinforced because it again helped you stay away from the dreaded thief.

During treatment sessions, negative reinforcers are not used frequently. Therefore, we will concentrate on positive reinforcers. Remember, though that negative reinforcement is not punishment. A rate of response decreases under punishment but increases under negative reinforcement.

Food and drink are the main **positive primary reinforcers**. In some cases, a response followed by food may be learned faster. It is often pointed out that food is an unnatural reinforcer for communicative behaviors. When a little girl correctly names the family dog the first time, no one puts some apple sauce in her mouth. This is true and yet you should know that some communicative behaviors are reinforced primarily. For these behaviors, only the primary reinforcers will do. For example, when you ask for a glass of water, only a glass of water or some kind of drink will do. All your requests for food and drink are reinforced primarily. Therefore, it is not correct to say that speech and language behaviors are never primarily reinforced. It is correct to say that some speech and language behaviors are reinforced primarily and most are reinforced socially.

During treatment, clinicians use primary reinforcers because of clinical reasons, not because they are natural. Food and drink may be used when other, more natural events do not have an effect. The following guidelines suggest ways of using primary reinforcers.

1. Use food and drink only when other reinforcers do not work. Expect to use them with infants, and persons who are nonverbal and profoundly retarded.

2. Before selecting primary reinforcers, discuss it with the client, or more likely, with the family members. Consider their objections or recommendations regarding the kinds of food to use. Select healthy food items. Avoid foods that are not recommended for medical reasons.

3. Ask parents to withhold the reinforcers before coming to the session. Better yet, arrange treatment sessions around snack time or lunch time so that the infant or the child is motivated for your primary reinforcer.

4. Always use social reinforcers with primary reinforcers. For instance, praise the boy for the correct response as you let him have a sip of juice.

5. Eventually, fade the primary reinforcer and keep only the social reinforcers.

Social Reinforcers. Reinforcing effects of some events depend on past experiences. These events reinforce because of their association with other kinds of reinforcers. Events that reinforce because of past experiences are called **social reinforcers**. They also are called conditioned reinforcers.

Social reinforcers are natural reinforcers for many kinds of verbal responses. In everyday communication, social reinforcers are used frequently. Therefore, they are preferable in treatment sessions.

There are many specific events or stimuli that act as social reinforcers. In communication, attention to a speaker, a smile, a nod, a touch, a pat on the shoulder, verbal approval, verbal praise, and other kinds of verbal and nonverbal responses from the listener can be potential reinforcers. These are probably the most frequently used social reinforcers in treatment sessions.

As noted before, social reinforcers may not be effective with nonverbal clients, infants, and individuals who are profoundly retarded who may not have experienced the reinforcing value of verbal and other stimuli. Even so, some social stimuli may be effective. Infants respond to touch and smile. People who are profoundly retarded also may react to some of these stimuli.

You know that social reinforcers are used even when primary reinforcers are used. While primary reinforcers are withdrawn eventually, some level of social reinforcement is always maintained. This means that social reinforcers are used in all stages of treatment. Therefore, select and use social reinforcers according to the following guidelines.

1. With infants and clients who are profoundly retarded, use smile and touch along with primary reinforcers. Add praise and other verbal stimuli as they seem to gain reinforcing value for the client.
2. Use social reinforcers naturally. When you say "Good boy!" or "Excellent job!" or "I like that!" smile and show proper emotional expressions that go with such statements. You should sound and look happy when a correct response is produced. Use appropriate patterns of intonation so you do not sound like a robot when praising the client.

Conditioned Generalized Reinforcers. Certain events that have a more pervasive effect on behavior are called **conditioned generalized reinforcers**. These events become reinforcing because of their association with other reinforcers. In that respect, conditioned generalized reinforcers are similar to social reinforcers.

The two are different only in one respect. A conditioned generalized reinforcer can affect a response through several other events or objects that may be gained by it. An ordinary social reinforcer has to effect a change by its own power. For example, a token, which is a conditioned generalized reinforcer may be effective because it can be exchanged for a variety of other reinforcers. A token is not just a token. It can mean anything you say because it can be exchanged for many other reinforcers. But verbal praise is only verbal praise. Either it is effective or it is not.

You can use plastic chips for tokens that may be exchanged for other reinforcers the child chooses in a session. Similarly, check marks entered in a booklet or stars and stickers pasted on a sheet of paper, points accumulated, marbles given, and coins earned may be exchanged for chosen reinforcers. You can use anything as a token provided it is dispensed easily for correct responses and exchanged later for a reinforcer.

Because tokens are not effective by themselves, you should have a collection of reinforcers for which clients can exchange their tokens. A common mistake in using tokens is to not have a backup reinforcement system. This mistake is made because some children do seem to respond to tokens even when nothing is available for exchange. Some children happily collect plastic tokens that are not good for anything. Others seem to be content with stars pasted on a sheet of paper. Stickers are popular with many children. But these items may work for a while only because they have been naturally backed-up. That is, they have meant something to children: verbal praise, a treat from parents, a previous backup reinforcer of some sort. The clinician cannot capitalize on this forever. If you go on giving tokens without backups, the correct response rate is likely to decline. Sooner or later, you have to pay for it! You need backup reinforcers.

Tokens are the most flexible of the reinforcers. For the child who does not respond to juice, you can offer an opportunity to play if a certain number of tokens are earned. If this does not work, you can offer to read a story for the same tokens. You may offer still other choices for the child: a small toy, a piece of gum, a walk through the clinic with you. The limits of a backup system are only practical. Because of this flexibility and the resulting power of the conditioned generalized reinforcers, they are an excellent choice. Use them with the following guidelines.

1. Tokens can be expensive if you need to back them with toys and other gifts. Consider this before you design a token system. Your clinic may not have any funds to purchase backup reinforcers. Do not promise a child that the parents will back up your tokens unless the parents previously have agreed to it.

2. Always have some backup reinforcers.
3. Ask the child to choose the reinforcer at the beginning of the session.
4. Tell the child how many tokens are needed to receive the backup reinforcer.
5. Do not set the number of tokens too high. The child must be able to exchange tokens for the chosen backup. If not, all the correct responses given in the session may be technically unreinforced. Therefore, set a number the child is likely to achieve.
6. Do not always limit your backups to toys, food, and other tangibles. Such activities as reading a story to the child, working on a puzzle, or taking a walk on the campus may be just as effective while being more fun.

Feedback. Both adults and children wish to know how well they are doing in therapy. When that information is systematically given to them, their performance or movement toward a target may be reinforced. The information given back to a person or a mechanical system about how the person or the system has been performing is called feedback. **Feedback is a reinforcer** when it increases the rate of response or some quality of it.

Feedback became a powerful tool in changing behavior with the invention of mechanical feedback devices. These devices were especially helpful in giving information about neurophysiological activities that could not be readily observed. For example, without the help of a mechanical device, you cannot give feedback to a person about the electrical activity of muscles. Such information given back to a person about his or her neurophysiological activities through a mechanical device is called **biofeedback**.

Biofeedback is used in treating stuttering and voice disorders. Several mechanical devices are available to monitor phonatory onset, continuous phonation, and muscle tension. Several kinds of electronic units help reduce the rate of speech in stutterers by giving delayed auditory feedback of their speech. Electromyographic instruments help reduce a speaker's muscle tension.

Biofeedback has been successful especially in treating voice disorders. As mentioned earlier, such instruments as PM 100 Pitch Analyzer, the Phonatory Function Analyzer, and the Visi-Pitch give feedback to clients on their vocal pitch and their attempts at changing it. Nasal resonance problems may be altered by the Nasometer which displays a ratio of oral and nasal resonance. In gradual steps, the client can increase the ratio in favor of the target resonance.

Increased use of computers in treatment will make mechanical feedback more common in therapy. Yet, feedback given to clients in treatment need not be mechanical. You may tell a stuttering man that his rate of dysfluency in the previous 5 minutes of conversation was 15% compared to 17% in the previous session. You may inform a woman that her hoarseness has been reduced some 50% over the past three sessions. A boy in articulation treatment may learn that his correct production of /s/ has increased from 30 to 90%. Such information about the performance levels is feedback and when used systematically, it can increase the rate of responses.

Sophisticated computer programs that are becoming available will make the task of giving instantaneous feedback easier and more attractive. Many computer programs currently are available to give immediate feedback on various aspects of speech and voice production.

Feedback, whether mechanical or not, is an essential part of all treatment. Therefore, use it according to the following guidelines.

1. Always give informational feedback in a comparative manner. Say where the client was and how close the performance is to reaching the final target or some intermediate criterion of performance.
2. In working with children, show progress graphically. Use colors whenever practical. If available, use computers which colorfully display on their monitors the progress and movement toward the target.
3. Do not give feedback only at the end of a session. Give it throughout the session so you can make it contingent on responses.
4. Combine mechanical feedback with verbal praise.
5. Do not continue to give negative feedback when the client makes little or no progress. Something is not working right. Perhaps you should change the treatment procedure or further simplify the target response.

High Probability Behaviors. An interesting fact about behavior is that **one action of a person can reinforce (increase) another action of the same person**. The behavior that reinforces is of high probability. That is, it is exhibited frequently. The behavior that is reinforced (increased), is of low probability. It is exhibited infrequently. The unique aspect of high probability behaviors as reinforcers is that both the reinforcer and the reinforced are the behaviors of the same person.

In using high probability behaviors to reinforce low probability behaviors, the clinician does not give anything except an opportunity to perform that highly desired behavior. But that opportunity is given only when the client performs what he or she is not likely to perform. Thus, the clinician increases the frequency of an unlikely behavior.

Target communicative behaviors are of low probability. The goal of treatment is to increase their frequency. To do this, first you must find a behavior that the client exhibits frequently. Does the client frequently paint, sing, read, listen to music, ski, go to movies, or talk to friends on the phone? Can any of these actions be used to reinforce target communicative behaviors under treatment?

Some high probability activities can be allowed in the treatment session itself. You may give a child 2 or 3 minutes to read a brief story or a part of a story after a certain number of correct responses are given. Opportunities to draw or paint, put puzzles together, listen to a song played on a tape recorder are among other activities that can be used to reinforce target responses in the clinic.

Opportunities for other behaviors cannot be provided in the clinic. The child cannot ski or see a movie in the treatment room. Often, these are the behaviors of highest probability with the greatest reinforcement potential. These behaviors may occur days or weeks after treatment sessions in which the target responses are produced. High probability behaviors in such cases are at best delayed reinforcers.

To bridge the gap between the eventual high probability behavior and the target responses, use a token system. Reinforce each correct response with a token. Require a certain number of tokens to engage in that cherished behavior. Obviously, in case of children, you should have the approval of parents who will make such opportunities available. In case of adults, you should have some system to verify the client's compliance with the arrangement.

High probability behaviors are among the most powerful reinforcers. Therefore, whenever you can, use them according to the following guidelines.

1. In talking with parents and clients, always try to find potential high probability behaviors.
2. When you use one, find a way to control unauthorized opportunities for it. You do not have a reinforcer if the client gets to ski every weekend regardless of the number of tokens earned.
3. In the beginning, require a number of tokens that will assure the opportunity for the high probability behavior. Increase

the required number of tokens in gradual steps.

4. With young children, give brief but frequent breaks for the high probability behaviors.
5. Do not avoid using a behavior that takes extra time to complete. A longer story may be read in chunks. A complex puzzle may be completed in stages. Require a small number of tokens to read a few paragraphs or to fit a few pieces of the puzzle.

Instructions, modeling, shaping, and reinforcing consequences discussed so far help you create new responses and increase the frequency of new and existing responses. But to strengthen and sustain those responses, you need to use reinforcers in certain ways. Next we will discuss those procedures.

Strengthening and Sustaining Target Behaviors

To strengthen and sustain responses you shape or increase, you must use reinforcers differently in different stages of treatment. The pattern of reinforcement arranged for a pattern of responses is called **a schedule of reinforcement**. One kind of schedule must be used to create and increase responses and another kind to sustain and strengthen them.

In a **continuous schedule**, every response is reinforced. This schedule is necessary in the early stage of treatment when the response needs to be shaped or increased to a higher frequency. A continuous schedule is helpful in establishing a behavior, but not in sustaining it. A continuously reinforced response is susceptible to extinction when reinforcement is stopped. After the dismissal, the client may not maintain the target responses because of infrequent reinforcement or lack of it in the natural environment.

A paradoxical effect of reinforcement schedule is that responses are strengthened more when they are not reinforced continuously. On an **intermittent schedule**, some responses are reinforced and other responses go unreinforced. There are many patterns of reinforcement and nonreinforcement resulting in many intermittent schedules.

In a **fixed ratio** schedule, a response is reinforced after a fixed number of unreinforced responses have been made. For example, a fixed ratio of 10, abbreviated FR10 means that you reinforce every 10th response. This schedule creates a pattern of 9 unreinforced responses and a 10th reinforced response.

A fixed ratio schedule is easy to use and has been used frequently in clinical and educational work. After a period of continuous reinforcement to establish a target response, you should switch to a fixed ratio schedule. For example, you may initially reinforce a child continuously for naming a set of pictured stimuli. When the child's correct response rate increases substantially, say from 10 % to over 50%, you may shift to an intermittent schedule. Your first intermittent schedule may be an FR2 (every second response is reinforced). When the response rate shows a further, significant increase, you may switch the schedule again, perhaps to an FR5. A fixed ratio allows you to make a progressive reduction in the amount of reinforcement delivered for correct responses.

In a variable ratio schedule, the number of responses required before giving a reinforcer varies around an average. Compared to a fixed ratio of 5 in which every fifth response is reinforced, in a variable ratio of 5 (VR5), an average of 5 responses are required before a reinforcer is given. Because the schedule is based on an average, the actual number of responses required on any given occasion will vary. You may reinforce the 7th response on one occasion and the 3rd on the next.

The variable ratio is a systematic, predetermined way of reinforcing responses. It is not one that you randomly reinforce responses and then find out the average after the session is over. The variable ratio is determined beforehand and reinforcers are given in such a way as to conform to an average number of unreinforced responses. This is done most efficiently with electronic equipment that calculates the average from occasion to occasion and delivers the reinforcer automatically. When such an equipment is not available, you can prepare a schedule that varies around an average. In the session, you may have a sheet of paper that tells you to reinforce every 4th, 7th, 3rd, 9th, or 6th response.

Variable ratio produces a strong response rate. Whenever possible, use this schedule in the latter stages of treatment. Use a variable ratio schedule especially when you monitor the target behaviors in conversational speech.

Typically, a schedule specifies what behavior will be reinforced and how frequently. But there is an unusual schedule which specifies what behavior will not be reinforced. This schedule is called the **differential reinforcement of other behavior (DRO)**. Sometimes, what matters most is that a client not exhibit a certain behavior. In such cases, there is one or a few unacceptable behaviors but there are many acceptable behaviors that could be produced instead. So your schedule specifies what behavior or behaviors will not be reinforced. This means that many other alternate behaviors will be reinforced.

Suppose you are working with a small group of children and a boy in the group refuses to sit in his chair. He moves around and disturbs other children working on their assignments. In this case, not sitting in the chair is the troublesome behavior; instead the child could be reading, sitting quietly, working on his arithmetic, coloring, and so forth. Therefore, you tell the child that he will be reinforced provided that he does not leave the chair. You reinforce any of the desirable behaviors including just sitting in the chair.

Two other frequently discussed schedules are the fixed interval and the variable interval. While the ratio schedules are based on the number of responses that go unreinforced between reinforcers, the interval schedules are based on the time that lapses between reinforced responses. In a **fixed interval schedule (FI)**, an invariable period of time lapses between any two opportunities for presenting a reinforcer. In a **variable interval schedule (VI)**, the amount of time that lapses between two such opportunities is varied around an average.

An important thing to remember about the interval schedules is that the reinforcer is not automatically given after the specified fixed or variable time interval passes. The lapse of the interval creates an opportunity for reinforcement. The first response made after the interval is over is reinforced. That first response may or may not be made precisely at the end of the interval. Always remember that a reinforcer must be given immediately after a response is made.

Interval schedules have not been used frequently in treating communicative disorders though they have some potential. In treating voice and fluency disorders, you can use interval schedules. For example, a stuttering speaker's fluent speech may be reinforced on a VI10 s (variable interval of 10 seconds). In this schedule, you reinforce if the speaker maintains fluency during 10-second intervals on the average. Similarly, a speaker with hoarseness may be reinforced for clear voice on a fixed or variable time schedule.

How To Effectively Use Reinforcement Schedules. Generally, variable ratio and variable interval schedules produce stronger responses than fixed ratio or fixed interval schedules. But all intermittent schedules produce stronger response rates than the continuous schedule. Therefore, use the following guidelines in arranging reinforcement schedules.

1. Begin with continuous reinforcement. During response shaping and modeling, reinforce every correct response.
2. When nonimitated response rates show a substantial increase over baselines, switch to a fixed ratio schedule.
3. Start with a small ratio, perhaps an FR2.
4. Increase the ratio in small steps as the correct response rates continue to increase.
5. Use a large ratio during conversational speech. An FR10 or larger should work. If possible, use a variable interval ratio.
6. If a switch to a thinner schedule of reinforcement causes a decline in the correct response rate, lower the schedule.
7. Use DRO when many desirable behaviors are incompatible with one or a few undesirable behaviors.

Sequence of Treatment

Treatment is started after you have assessed the client's communicative behaviors and selected the target behaviors. However, before you begin treatment, you must establish baselines of target behaviors.

Baselines of Target Behaviors

Baselines show a client's pretreatment response rates. Baselines are necessary to assess the client's improvement with treatment. The client's progress may be judged continuously against the baselines.

The assessment data are not enough to evaluate the client improvement in treatment because the data may be dated by the time you start treatment. More importantly, measures of communicative behaviors taken during assessment are limited, not repeated, and hence of questionable reliability. Therefore, you need to establish baselines just before starting treatment to get current, reliable, and comprehensive data on the client's status before treatment.

In baserating behaviors, measures are repeated to establish reliability. For example, instead of taking one conversational speech sample to assess articulation, language features, or stuttering, you take two or more samples to find a somewhat stable rate of those behaviors. Because you can focus only on the immediate target responses, you can afford to take more extensive measures than it is possible during assessment. For example, during assessment, you wish to find out all phonemes in error; having already known this, during baserating, you measure in depth only a few of the misarticulated phonemes targeted for immediate treatment. You baserate new phonemes when you are ready to teach them. This method always gives you both reliable and current pretreatment response rates.

To obtain comprehensive baselines, responses should be sampled adequately. For example, it is not sufficient to give one or two opportunities to produce a phoneme or a grammatical morpheme. Typically, this is all a standardized test can do. Therefore, you must prepare an adequate number of stimulus materials to evoke the target responses on repeated trials. For baserating speech and language targets, roughly 20 stimulus items are needed to measure the production of target responses. When combined with repeated speech and language samples, such measures reflect pretreatment response rates more accurately than test results.

How To Baserate Target Behaviors. Use the following guidelines to baserate target behaviors.

1. Baserate only those behaviors that you plan to teach immediately. Repeat a baseline before teaching any behavior, even if it was baserated a few weeks earlier. Because behaviors tend to change, only a baseline taken just prior to treatment is valid.
2. Write instructions to the client. Also, write questions to evoke the target responses. You need questions to evoke responses to pictured stimuli. Select physical stimuli (pictures or objects).
3. Plan how you might take conversational speech samples. To sample language structures adequately, you should direct conversation so that opportunities for producing infrequently used language structures are presented. See Appendix D for guidelines on taking and analyzing language samples.
4. For an articulation or language client, write at least 20 response exemplars for each target behavior. An exemplar may be a word, phrase, or sentence that contains a target response. For instance, the word *soup* or the phrase *hot soup* or the sentence *I like soup* contains the /s/, a potential target response for a child who misarticulates it. Each of those three is an exemplar. Similarly, in teaching the present progressive *ing*,

you might have such exemplars as *walking, boy walking,* and *boy is walking,* and so forth. Your exemplars may be of one kind only. You may have 20 words, phrases, or sentences depending on the initial level of training. They are likely to be words or phrases.

5. Present the 20 stimulus items on discrete trials. A discrete trial gives the client one opportunity to produce the target response. Typically, you show the picture or object, ask a question, and wait for the response. Also, baserate imitative responses on a set of trials in which you model the responses after asking the question.

6. Take an adequate conversational speech sample. Ask the client or parents to bring taped conversational speech samples from home to assess the target behavior rate in extraclinical situations.

7. Record each response on a recording sheet. See Appendix P for a sample discrete trial baseline recording sheet.

8. In case of articulation and language clients, calculate the percentage correct response rate separately for discrete trials and for the conversational speech samples. Also, calculate the response rates separately for clinical speech samples and home samples. For fluency clients, calculate the percentage dysfluency rates based on the number of words spoken. For voice clients, you may calculate durations of conversational speech that are free of problems and those durations that are characterized by such problems as hoarseness or nasality.

9. If any two measures for the same response mode and situation are not comparable, repeat the measures. For instance, if two clinic speech samples show different baselines, then you need to repeat them. Similarly, if two home samples disagree widely, you need additional home samples. Home and clinic samples may vary in case of stuttering and voice characteristics. But the response rates should not vary much in case of articulation and language.

10. Write objective statements to summarize the baseline data. Such objective statements help evaluate the effects of subsequent treatment by giving a quantitative specification of the client's status before treatment:

The child's correct articulation of /s/ in conversational speech, measured across three samples, was 20%. Each sample contained at least 10 opportunities to produce the phoneme.

The client's rate of dysfluency on two home samples of at least 2,000 words each was 13 and 15%.

The client's longest fluent utterances, measured over two conversational speech samples of 800 words each, typically lasted 10 seconds. (Note: this is a durational baserate of fluency. The measure is a statistical mode—which is the most frequently occurring event—not an average.)

The client's voice was judged hypernasal on 90% of utterances that did not contain nasal speech.

The client was hoarse 90% of the time she spoke during two baserate sessions. She spoke at least 500 words or more in each session. (Note: another durational baserate measure.)

The patient did not recall the names of 5 of his close relatives including his wife. The patient was asked to name them on three occasions each separated by 24 hours.

Ten per cent of the words spoken by the patient were jargon.

The Table 1 shows the correct production of seven grammatic morphemes recorded across three samples. (You can present data in tabular form. In this case, you list the grammatic morphemes and the percentage correct production rate for each of them. A similar table may be prepared for a client's multiple misarticulations.)

The Initial Treatment Sequence

The Number of Target Behaviors. After establishing baselines, begin teaching the target behaviors. The first question you face is: How many behaviors can I teach in individual sessions? There is no single rule that you can follow in all cases. Much depends on the disorder of the client, severity of the disorder, the general learning ability of the person, age, education, and other subject characteristics. But equally important are the clinician's expertise, the duration of sessions, and whether the client is treated individually or in a group.

To start with, try the following recommendations; if they do not work, you should analyze the data to find out what went wrong.

1. Be ready to initiate training on three to five phonemes in syllables or words.
2. Plan on initiating training on two to four grammatical morphemes, syntactic structures, and other language features.

3. Be prepared to instruct and model all the basic skills of fluency in the first full session of treatment. If the session lasts at least 30 minutes, you should be able to go over the skills and initiate practice on all of them. In the case of persons who learn fast, you may be able to move from the single-word level to two-word phrases or even to short sentences in one or two sessions.

4. Expect to instruct and model the target behaviors and initiate training on voice targets in the first treatment session. If you use a feedback instrument, be ready to fully demonstrate it and start training the client on it. Depending on the client's learning rate, you may be able to move from word to phrases and sentences in the first session or two.

Structure of Treatment Sessions. The argument you often hear about tight versus loose structure of treatment sessions is not that important. Like every other aspect of treatment, the structure of individual sessions is also client-specific. Use the tight structure if the client needs it, use the loose structure if the client can handle it. If the client is able to learn language structures in an informal conversational format, start treatment in that format. Obviously, to do this, the child should have enough language skills to carry on a conversation. Typically, such children need to learn only a few and perhaps advanced language structures.

The client who is minimally verbal or nonverbal, or has multiple misarticulations, often responds better under a structured format. The technical advantage of the structured discrete trial format is that it allows you to evoke many more target responses than it is possible in such loose formats as the incidental teaching procedure. In this latter procedure, you wait for the child to initiate conversation and reinforce language productions as they are made by the child in the normal process of interaction. With most children who are moderate to severely impaired, this arrangement can work efficiently in the latter stages of treatment. Actually, in the final stages of treatment, this should be the format for most if not all clients.

Instead of seeing tight versus loose structure as either/or options, see them as a matter of sequence. Initially therapy is more structured, but only as structured as it needs to be. Therapy may be highly structured in some cases, less so in others, and not at all in some. Gradually, the tight structure is faded so that the treatment situation comes to resemble everyday communicative interaction.

Discrete Trial Procedure. The initial training is better started with some structure especially when the targets are narrowly defined articulation and language targets. Therefore, in most cases, use the structured discrete trial procedure to establish the target speech and language responses. The discrete trials are less useful or not at all needed in treating fluency and voice problems.

Steps in administering discrete treatment trials are described in Appendix P. In the treatment of articulation and language disorders, a discrete trial consists of (1) stimulus presentation; (2) asking a question that normally evokes the target response; (3) modeling; (4) giving a few seconds for the client to respond; (5) consequating the response; (6) recording the response; (7) marking the end of the trial by pulling the stimulus away; and, (8) starting the next trial after a few seconds.

Practice the stimulus presentation so that you can administer each trial quickly and efficiently. Instruct, ask questions, and model responses as described earlier. In consequating responses, make a quick judgment about the accuracy of the client responses. If the response is correct, immediately reinforce it. If it is wrong, use one of the response reduction procedures described in Chapter 8. Record every response of the client on a recording sheet. (See Appendix K for a sample.)

Movement Through the Treatment Sequence

When the treatment is working, you will see systematic increase in the client's target behaviors. As this happens, you begin to make important clinical decisions. To take a client from the initial imitation of a narrowly defined target response to the final stage of conversational speech in natural settings, you must move from one stage of treatment to the next.

Each movement is progress. But each movement requires a clinical decision. A wrong decision made at a juncture point might retard the client progress. For example, if you spent too much time reinforcing the isolated production of a phoneme, it may be difficult for you to move the client on to the word level of training. The following general guidelines should help you make decisions to move to a different level of training. The guidelines are also clinical criteria of movement through stages of treatment.

Criteria for Clinical Decisions

When Do I Stop or Reinstate Modeling?

1. **Stop modeling** when the client imitates the initial target response on at least five consecutive trials.
2. **Reinstate modeling** when you observe incorrect responses

on three to four trials with no modeling. Again, stop modeling after five correctly imitated responses. If you have to stop and reinstate modeling repeatedly, continue modeling until the client gives 10 or more imitated responses. Alternately, see if the client can give correct responses if you continued a little longer without modeling.

Training Criteria for Target Response vs. Behaviors. To understand some of the subsequent criteria, you should make a **distinction between a target response and a target behavior**. As you know, you use some 20 words in teaching a phoneme. The production of each word that contains the target phoneme is a target response; the correct production of the phoneme in varied contexts and in conversational speech is the target behavior. Likewise, in teaching a grammatical morpheme, you may have some 20 or so sentences that contain that target morpheme. The production of each sentence is a target response; the production of the morpheme in varied contexts and in conversational speech is the target behavior.

Earlier we discussed exemplars. Each specific response is an exemplar of the target behavior. The word *soup* is an exemplar of /s/ (or another phoneme in it). The word *walking* is an exemplar of the present progressive. Production of the phoneme /s/ and the present progressive are target behaviors.

When we say that a client has multiple articulation targets to learn, we do not mean the 20 or so sentences for each phoneme; we mean the number of phonemes to be taught. Similarly, when we say the child has multiple grammatic morphemes to learn, we do not mean any particular word or sentence that contains a morpheme; we mean such classes of responses as the regular plural, present progressive, an article, a preposition, and so forth.

You also can think of a target behavior as a group of similar responses and a target response as any one of those responses. We teach the more concrete individual responses to have the client master the more abstract target behavior.

When Is a Target Response Tentatively Trained?

A **target response** is tentatively trained when the client gives at least 10 consecutively correct, nonimitated responses. Suppose you were teaching a child the present progressive *ing* in words. Perhaps you were teaching four words with the target feature in it. When the child correctly produces the word *walking* 10 times in a row, you could consider that response (not the behavior) to have been tentatively learned.

Extend this logic to (1) a child under articulation training; and (2) a man under voice therapy who is being trained to say individual words without nasal resonance.

Explanation of the Criterion: This is a highly tentative criterion. Much work needs to be done to complete the teaching of the target behavior, but the client has met a tentative training criterion on one exemplar (response). You should stop training an exemplar at some point, and this is a suggested point. You can redefine this criterion just as appropriately as 15 or 20 consecutively correct responses.

When Is a Target Behavior Tentatively Trained?

A target behavior is tentatively trained when the client meets a tentative probe criterion of at least 90% correct response rate on probe trials. The tentative training criterion for a target behavior is based on an external procedure. That is, you cannot decide that a behavior (the /s/, the present progressive, oral resonance, normal voice quality) is tentatively trained because the responses on selected training words or phrases have been correct.

The Probe Procedure. To find out if the behavior meets the probe criterion, conduct probes. A probe is a procedure to find out if a trained response is produced on the basis of generalization. For example, a phoneme trained in a few words may be correctly produced in other, untrained words. A grammatic morpheme trained in a few sentences may be produced in other, untrained sentences. To say that a behavior is tentatively trained, you must document this generalized production.

Hold a probe when you have trained four to six target responses (e.g, four words or phrases). You may probe through discrete trials or speech samples. On **discrete trial probes**, you alternate the trained and the untrained stimuli. For example, of the 20 words you had baserated for teaching /s/ in words, assume that you have used four words in training. The client has met the tentative training criterion on each of those words. Now you probe to see if /s/ is tentatively trained. First, prepare a probe list on which the first is the one already trained. The second should be one of the words not used in training. The third is again a trained word, followed by an untrained word. Reuse the trained words until all the untrained words have been alternated with them.

Do not model any words. Show pictures to have the child name them or ask the child to read the printed words on the probe list. Reinforce the correct production of the trained words as you will have done on training trials; do not consequate in any way the right or wrong productions of the probe words.

Count the number of correct productions of untrained words only; ignore productions of trained words. Calculate the percentage of correct untrained word productions. This is your probe response rate. If this is at least 90%, you may assume that the target behavior has been tentatively trained.

Tape record a brief conversational speech sample making sure that at least 20 opportunities were available for producing the target behavior. Count how many were correctly produced. Calculate the percent correct probe rate for the conversational speech to see if it meets the criterion.

Use the same probe criterion at the level of words, phrases, or sentences. When you have completed training in sentences, use only the conversational speech probe to calculate the percent correct probe response rate.

Note that a behavior is trained only when some untrained exemplars of that behavior are produced correctly. You can use the same procedure to probe various language targets. For clients who stutter or those who have voice problems, probes should be conducted at the relevant level of response topography (phrases, sentences, conversational speech). Record the responses without consequating any of the behaviors. Measure the target behaviors of interest in the same way you did during baserate sessions. Calculate the percentage of probe response rates (e.g., percentage dysfluency rate or the percentage of utterances without hoarseness) and compare them against the percentages recorded during baserate sessions. Appendix G shows a sample probe recording sheet.

When Do I Make Topographical Shifts in Training?

Topographical shifts are made when you move to words from syllables, to phrases from words, and to sentences from words. These topographical shifts are necessary in the treatment of most disorders of communication.

It is likely that in most cases, you will have started training on three or four behaviors. The initial topographical level of training on most if not all of these behaviors may be syllables or words. The level is rarely conversational speech. But the final topographical level is always conversational speech.

The progress on multiple target behaviors under training is likely to vary. Each behavior is shaped through its own topographic sequence. One behavior may move through fewer sequences than the other. Some behaviors will meet the tentative training criterion sooner than others.

Make the first topographic shift when a behavior meets the tentative probe criterion at the initial response level. For example, when the initial probe shows 90% correct production of /s/ in untrained words, shift training to phrase level. When the phoneme production is 90% on probe phrases, shift to sentences. When the probe for sentences shows 90% correct, move to more natural conversational speech. Move again to more natural settings when within the clinic, the target phoneme is produced at 90% accuracy on conversational probes.

When one of the target behaviors meets the final criterion or any time you have extra treatment time, select another behavior for training. Start with a simple topography and move through a sequence.

Design a similar or modified sequence to training language features, fluency, and voice characteristics. Note that the probe criterion may be higher for fluency. Generally, 90% fluency is too low. A probe criterion of 97 or 98% is desirable.

What Do I Do When Probe Criteria Are Not Met?

A client may fail the probe criterion at any level of training. When this happens, give additional training at the same level. For example, the child who fails the tentative probe criterion at the word level of a phoneme training should be trained on new exemplars. Teach two to four new exemplars before you probe again. In some cases, especially when you already have trained 8 to 10 exemplars, a few additional training trials on all of the trained exemplars may be sufficient to have the client meet the probe criterion.

When Is a Target Behavior Finally Trained?

A target behavior finally is trained when its production in conversational speech in natural settings is acceptable. Different criteria may apply to different communicative behaviors. Phonemes and language structures may be considered finally trained when they are produced in conversational speech at 90% accuracy. Fluency may be considered trained when the client's rate of dysfluencies in conversational speech in extraclinical situations does not exceed 3 or 4%. Normal voice characteristics may be considered trained when they are sustained at least 90 or 95% of utterances or of speaking time.

The target behavior finally is trained when the client is ready for dismissal. You dismiss the client from services only when the communicative behaviors are produced under natural conditions.

The various criteria described so far are suggested guidelines for making clinical decisions. They have worked in clinical research. But always remember that no criterion is a rule you cannot violate and all criteria depend on the client performance. Design your criteria that are supported by clinical data. Each client's response rates you record are your clinical data. These data are your ultimate guiding principles.

8

Controlling Undesirable Behaviors

I n Chapter 7, one of the treatment tasks described was to reduce the frequency of undesirable behaviors. While implementing procedures to increase desirable communicative behaviors, you may use procedures that reduce undesirable communicative responses. In many cases, you also must reduce undesirable general behaviors that interfere with treatment.

Often, undesirable communicative behaviors are the ones the client or the parents complain about. They are the behaviors that need to be replaced by appropriate communicative behaviors.

Behaviors To Be Reduced

Reduce the following undesirable communicative behaviors while working with your clients.

1. **Disorders of Language.** Undesirable communicative behaviors to be reduced in clients with language disorders include, among others, gesturing, crying or fussing when something is wanted, using inappropriate words or semantic,

203

syntactic, and morphologic features, and inappropriate use of language in social situations.

2. **Articulation and phonological disorders.** Misarticulation of isolated speech sounds or patterns of misartculations are the behaviors to be reduced.

3. **Voice disorders.** The behaviors to be reduced include breathiness, hoarseness, harshness, inappropriate pitch or loudness, hyper- or hyponasality, hard glottal attacks, and vocally abusive behaviors.

4. **Disorders of fluency.** In the initial stages of stuttering treatment, behaviors to be reduced include dysfluencies, speech rate, abrupt initiation of sound, inappropriate management of airflow, muscular tension associated with speech production, and avoidance of words and speaking situations. In the latter stages of treatment, you need to reduce monotonous and excessively slow speech that was targeted in the initial stages. In treating persons with cluttering, you need to reduce dysfluencies, imprecise articulation, excessively fast rate of speech, and poor organization or formulation of sentences.

You will encounter a wide array of undesirable general behaviors that interfere with treatment process. **Among others, you should reduce behaviors of the following type.**

1. **Inattentive behaviors.** Especially a problem with children, inattentive and distractible behaviors interfere with treatment. Unless these behaviors are reduced, treatment cannot be focused on the desirable target behaviors.

2. **Crying, fussing, and other emotionally laden behaviors.** These are among the strong disruptors of the treatment process. They can be emotionally upsetting to the clinician who does not know how to handle them.

3. **Out-of-seat and other uncooperative behaviors.** Children who begin to move around in the therapy room, crawl under the table, or simply wiggle around in their seats cannot focus on treatment targets.

4. **Absenteeism.** A larger problem is a no show or frequent cancellations of treatment sessions. Obviously, clients who do not attend treatment sessions cannot be helped.

5. **General unresponsivity.** Many clients show a generalized unresponsivity to treatment. Stimuli and treatment processes

do not interest them. In such cases, lack of motivation for responding and working with the clinician seem to be the main problems that interfere with the treatment process.

Many clients interweave undesirable behaviors with appropriate responses. The undesirable communicative behaviors, such as the undifferentiated gestures of the nonverbal and the speech sound errors of a child with misarticulations may be more frequent in the beginning but decline as treatment proceeds. Probably the best way of reducing undesirable communicative behaviors is to increase the desirable counterparts. For instance, the most effective way of reducing misarticulations is to increase correct productions of speech sounds.

Undesirable general behaviors that interfere with treatment often need some special procedures. An occasional interfering behavior is not a serious problem. At times, children wiggle in their chairs and fail to pay attention to the stimuli presented. These may be controlled easily by instructions and reinforcement. But when the client consistently exhibits interfering behaviors, you must take special steps.

How To Find Out the Maintaining Causes of Undesirable Behaviors

If you can assess the potential maintaining causes of an undesirable behavior, you can reduce or eliminate them more efficiently. It may not always be possible to find out what maintains undesirable (or desirable) behaviors. It is difficult to say how stuttering, misarticulations, and inappropriate or inadequate language, and voice quality deviations are maintained. Similarly, it is often not clear why the child is crying, wiggling in the chair, or exhibiting other interfering behaviors.

You can take some steps prior to starting treatment to find out potential maintaining variables. While establishing baselines, you may introduce the variable you suspect is maintaining an undesirable behavior to see what happens. Baselines that also are used to find out the maintaining causes of behaviors being measured are called **functional analysis baselines** (Mason & Iwata, 1990). A functional analysis helps you determine causes of behaviors.

In hindsight, successful treatment sometimes tells you what maintained an undesirable behavior. For example, you may find out that a nonverbal child's undifferentiated gestural or vocal attempts at communication have decreased after learning useful and effective verbal communication. A child who can request something in words is less likely to cry, fuss, or point to things wanted. In such a case, you might think that parental reinforcement maintained the undifferentiated attempts at communication.

In applied behavioral analysis, scientists have made systematic attempts at finding maintaining causes of some interfering behaviors. For example, studies of experimental analysis of self-injurious or self-stimulatory behaviors have suggested that these and possibly other undesirable behaviors may be maintained by either positive reinforcement, negative reinforcement, or automatic reinforcement (Durand & Carr, 1987; Iwata, Pace, Kalsher, Cowdery, & Cataldo, 1990; Repp, Felce, & Barton, 1988).

Most often, **attention** is the positive reinforcer that maintains undesirable behaviors. A teacher who otherwise ignored a child may promptly attend to a child's misbehavior, thus inadvertently reinforcing the troublesome behavior. These behaviors are most effectively reduced by extinction (withholding attention).

To find out if an undesirable behavior is maintained by positive reinforcement, while measuring the frequency of the behavior prior to treatment, you may pay attention to it to see if the frequency of the behavior increases. You can then withdraw attention to see if the frequency of the behavior decreases. If the behavior increases as you pay attention and decreases as you ignore it, then the behavior is most likely maintained by positive reinforcement.

Negative reinforcement maintains an undesirable behavior when that behavior terminates an aversive event. For example, a child, faced with a difficult task demand (an aversive event), may exhibit an undesirable behavior (Weeks & Gaylord-Ross, 1981). Observing this behavior, the clinician may stop making those demands. In this case, the child escaped from the difficult task by exhibiting an undesirable behavior. This is negative reinforcement. One way of reducing such negatively reinforced undesirable behaviors is to prevent escape by not terminating the task demand. The clinician should continue to make the demands and reinforce compliance.

To find out if an undesirable behavior is maintained by negative reinforcement, you can present some difficult tasks and see if the behavior increases in frequency. If it does, the behavior most likely is maintained by negative reinforcement. For example, you might present a series of trials on which a nonverbal child who frequently exhibits undesirable behaviors is asked to imitate relatively long and unusual words, a difficult task for the child. Having failed to give correct responses on repeated trials, the child may begin to exhibit the undesirable behavior (e. g., leaving the chair, crawling under the table). These behaviors are the child's way of escaping from a difficult (hence aversive) task demand. The escape negatively reinforces the behaviors.

Automatic reinforcement is presumed when behaviors do not seem to have environmentally generated maintaining causes. Neither externally delivered positive reinforcement nor negative reinforcement seems to account for the frequency of the behavior under observation. Therefore, undesirable behaviors are presumed to generate **neural consequences of reinforcement**. Lack of stimulation and activity frequently are cited reasons for undesirable behaviors that are maintained by automatic reinforcement. In these children, providing opportunities for play and other kinds of activities, manipulation and exploration of toys and other materials tend to reduce their undesirable behaviors.

To find out if undesirable behaviors are maintained by automatic reinforcement, you need to leave the child alone in a room and see if the behaviors occur. Automatic reinforcement is most often presumed in case of stereotypic or self-stimulatory behaviors. An autistic boy may rock himself endlessly when left alone. It is difficult to point out positive or negative reinforcement for such behaviors. A reasonable assumption is that such self-stimulatory behaviors generate their own neural consequences that are reinforcing.

General Strategies for Decreasing Undesirable Behaviors

Procedures that reduce behaviors make no distinction between desirable and undesirable or good and bad behaviors. Behaviors are so described from a personal and social viewpoint. Procedures that decrease behaviors may decrease any behavior: desirable, undesirable, good, or bad. Therefore, the prudent clinician's job is to apply response reduction procedures to only the undesirable behaviors.

Most textbooks on behavioral treatment procedures classify response reduction procedures as extinction and punishment. Several procedures typically described under extinction and various forms of punishment are included here and are considered appropriate for therapeutic use. Behavior therapists have repeatedly emphasized that the scientific and therapeutic meaning of punishment does not share the negative connotations of punishment in everyday language. Nonetheless, we wish to minimize the use of the term punishment because its scientific meaning constantly is confused with its everyday meaning of a collection of many painful, exploitative, and vain procedures. Also, the response reduction procedures recommended here do not include all of the punishment procedures researched in behavioral analysis. Therefore, we have taken a more descriptive approach in classifying response reduction procedures that you may use in clinical treatment.

We have classified the response reduction strategies as either direct or indirect. This classification depends on whether a treatment contingency is placed on the behavior to be reduced or on another behavior. In the **direct response reduction strategy**, you place a contingency on the behavior to be reduced. Obviously, you use a contingency that reduces the rate of responses. In the **indirect strategy**, you place a contingency on a desirable behavior whose increase will have an indirect effect of decreasing an undesirable behavior. Note that the behavior to be reduced is not directly manipulated. Also, you use a contingency that increases a behavior. An important point to remember is that an undesirable behavior may be reduced by increasing a desirable behavior.

Another important point to remember is that only direct response reduction procedures may be defined as those that reduce behaviors. Though indirect procedures also help us reduce behaviors, they are not response reduction procedures. The indirect procedures increase responses; they are reinforcement procedures. You should not say that we use reinforcement procedures to decrease behaviors. By definition, reinforcement procedures increase behaviors. When used in a program of response reduction, the reinforcement procedures increase desirable behaviors. Presumably, this makes the undesirable behavior unnecessary. This is an important reason for classifying some response reduction strategies as indirect.

In the following sections, we will return to this distinction to make it clearer to you. Specific procedures and examples will show how a contingency is placed either on the behavior to be reduced or on a different behavior to be increased.

Direct Strategy for Decreasing Behaviors

In the direct strategy, you concentrate on an undesirable behavior and place a contingency on it. The effect of this contingency is to directly reduce that behavior.

There are several procedures in which the behavior is directly reduced. These procedures fall into two major categories: stimulus presentation and stimulus withdrawal. We will describe specific procedures under these categories.

Stimulus Presentation

Responses may be reduced by **presenting a stimulus immediately after a response is made**. Research has shown that several response-contingent stimuli can reduce behaviors. When they do, the stimuli typically are considered punishing. Punishing stimuli are those that reduce the future probability of a behavior.

Verbal stimuli most frequently are used in reducing behaviors. Such verbal stimuli as "No," "Wrong," and "Not correct," have been shown to reduce behaviors if presented immediately after the production of an incorrect response. Most clinicians indicate to the client in some way that a given attempt to produce the target response was not acceptable. The indication may be more or less subtle. The clinician may shake his or her head in a disapproving manner, show other facial or hand gestures of disapproval, or use explicit verbal stimuli. In all cases, the clinician will have used stimulus presentation as the method of reducing the undesirable response.

By themselves, verbal stimuli may not be effective. However, when combined with strong reinforcers for desirable behaviors that are shaped in carefully designed incremental steps, verbal stimuli may be sufficient to reduce undesirable behaviors. If you did not use verbal or gestural means of saying that the response was not correct or fully acceptable, the client's incorrect responses may persist.

How To Use Stimulus Presentation. In using stimulus presentation as the method of response reduction, follow these suggestions.

1. **Present the verbal stimulus immediately after the response is made.** To do this, you must make quick evaluations of the correctness of client responses.
2. **Present the verbal stimulus in a firm and objective manner.** Say "No" in such a way that you mean it. You should not sound unsure. The message, not necessarily the voice, must be clear and loud.
3. **Though you say disapproving words, do not say them in angry manner.** You should not give an emotional response

to the incorrect response. Your tone should be objective and devoid of emotionality.

4. **Vary the words you use.** Do not use the same "No" or "Wrong" throughout an entire session.

Several other stimuli also may be used. When you take your clients to naturalistic settings during the maintenance stage of treatment, a mere touch on the arm may signal that a wrong response was made. In treatment sessions, stutterers often have been presented with white noise through headphones. Noise is known to reduce stuttering, though the reduction may be only temporary. In most clinical sessions, response reducing verbal stimuli are probably the most practical of all stimuli that may be presented response contingently.

Stimulus Withdrawal

Immediately after a response is made, you may **withdraw a stimulus that presumably strengthens, maintains, or increases that response.** While you present stimuli that weaken a response, you withdraw stimuli that reinforce it. In reducing responses, stimulus withdrawal may be more effective than stimulus presentation.

There are three specific procedures of stimulus withdrawal: time-out, response cost, and extinction. In all three, reinforcing events or consequences are withdrawn or made unavailable.

Time-Out. A frequently used method of behavior reduction is time-out from reinforcement. Time-out is a period of time during which all reinforcing events are suspended response contingently, and as a result, there typically is a decrease in the rate of that response.

The clinically useful forms of time-out include exclusion and nonexclusion time-out. In **exclusion time-out**, the child is excluded from the current setting and the activities. For example, you might ask a child to sit in the corner the instant he or she exhibits an undesirable behavior. All activities are terminated; the child is told to sit quietly. In this case, the setting is changed from the regular seating place to the corner. This is exclusion time-out.

In **nonexclusion time-out**, an undesirable behavior is followed immediately by cessation of all activity, but there is no physical movement and there is no change in the setting. For example, in stuttering treatment, you signal the client to stop talking for 5 seconds as soon as you observe a dysfluency or stutter. You avoid eye contact for the duration. At the end of the duration, you signal the person to resume talking. In this case, it is presumed that talking is reinforcing and interruption and silence are aversive. This aversive consequence is the presumed punisher that reduces the behavior on which it is made contingent. As you can see, <u>exclusion time-out is time-out from the ongoing activity; the activity is the presumed reinforcer; the person is not removed from the immediate setting.</u>

Many research studies have shown that time-out can reduce several forms of undesirable behavior. Unfortunately, time-out is also most often misused. Careless use of time-out may have a paradoxical effect on behavior: the behavior might increase in frequency. This is likely to happen when the time-in period and setting are not reinforcing and the time-out duration and setting are. Time-out may increase the undesirable behavior under the following conditions.

1. **Time-out provides unintended negative reinforcement.** An uncooperative behavior may bring relief from aversive treatment trials. For instance, as soon as fussing begins, you send the child to the corner. But this action terminated treatment trials (just what the child ordered, one might say). Consequently, the child's fussing behavior is negatively reinforced. When you resume treatment trials, the child may exhibit the undesirable behavior with added strength because this is how he or she can terminate treatment trials.

    <u>Treatment may be aversive because the (a) target behaviors are too difficult for the child, or (b) selected positive reinforcers given for the desirable behaviors are not working as such.</u> The desirable behaviors are not increasing and you say "No" to the child all too frequently because of the wrong responses.

2. **Time-out provides unintended positive reinforcement.** During time-out, the child may pull a small toy from his or her pocket and begin to play. A picture on the wall may provide positive reinforcement when you send the child to a corner. When asked to sit outside a classroom or treatment room, the child may enjoy people walking by or some activity going on outside. These events may positively reinforce the child's undesirable behavior because it is only through those behaviors that the child gets to watch outside activities. As soon as treatment is resumed, you may see an especially strong display of the undesirable behavior. Obviously, this troublesome behavior is the ticket to outside fun.

How To Use Time-out. Prudently and sparingly used, time-out has many advantages. Compared to several other response reduction procedures, time-out is only mildly aversive. It is not a difficult procedure to learn and use. Brief time-out periods do not waste much teaching time. Therefore, consider using time-out to reduce undesirable behaviors in your client. Use the following guidelines in developing an effective and safe time-out procedure.

1. **Avoid too brief or too long durations of time-out.** Durations that are too long may be ineffective because they may allow opportunities for other behaviors and take valuable time away from treatment. An appropriate duration depends on the nature of the behavior to be reduced. In reducing stuttering, for example, 5- to 10-second durations may be effective; longer durations are unnecessary. In controlling more global uncooperative, destructive, or inattentive behaviors, longer durations may be necessary. In most speech and language treatment sessions, the duration would not exceed 5 minutes.

2. **Try to avoid exclusion time-out as it is the least desirable procedure.** Do not use it unless you have tried nonexclusion time-out, extinction, response cost, and other procedures first and have found them ineffective.

3. **Signal the beginning of the nonexclusion time-out with a stimulus**. For example, you may raise your index finger to signal to a stuttering person that the 10-second time-out is started and that the speech must be terminated. In exclusion time-out, a young child may be guided physically to a time-out area without any signal. But in all cases, either a verbal statement or a nonhuman sound such as a buzzer should announce the end of the time-out period.

4. **Try to avoid physical contact in administering exclusion time-out.** If the child will comply with your instruction to go to the time-out area, do not use physical contact. Ask the child to go to the designated area and stay there until the end of the time-out period. Physically guide the child to the area only when the child does not comply.

5. **Use time-out on a continuous schedule.** Impose time-out on every instance of an undesirable behavior. Do not use an intermittent schedule, especially in the beginning of the response reduction program. Intermittent schedule may be useful in later stages of training when the undesirable behavior is of low frequency and you wish to keep it that way.

6. **Remove all reinforcers from the time-out area.** When you

use exclusion time-out, the area to which you send the child to spend the time-out duration should not contain reinforcing objects, people, and events. For instance, do not ask the child to sit in a hallway full of people and events. Failure to follow this rule is the main reason why sending a child to his or her own room for misbehaving usually is ineffective. Typically, the child's room is full of reinforcers.

7. **Release the client from time-out only when the undesirable behavior has been stopped.** If the child is still fussing in the corner, extend the time-out duration until the child becomes calm.

8. **Enrich the treatment situation with powerful and varied reinforcers.** Time-out is more effective when the return to the teaching situation is highly reinforcing and the time-out situation is dreary and unreinforcing. You will be in serious trouble if the situations are reversed.

Note that time-out will not reduce all behaviors in all clients. Besides, you should constantly watch for paradoxical effects. When you observe even a slight increase in the undesirable behavior being subjected to time-out, you should find an alternative procedure to reduce that behavior.

Response Cost. **Response cost** is a procedure of reducing behaviors through response contingent withdrawal of reinforcers. The client must give up a reinforcer every time an undesirable response is made.

Time-out and response cost are similar in that both deprive the client of some reinforcers. But their procedures are different. In time-out, you arrange a brief duration of no reinforcement of any kind; during this time, there is no responding; the person may even be moved from the behaving scene to another scene lacking reinforcers. In response cost, you take away a specific, tangible, reinforcer the client has earned or has been given; there is no particular interruption of responses; the client does not move physically.

Response cost is implemented most effectively and efficiently in a token system. Tokens are presented and withdrawn depending on the behavior. At the end of a treatment session, the remaining tokens are exchanged for a back-up reinforcer.

Response cost may be either the lose-only type or earn-and-lose type. In the **lose-only** type, you give the client a certain number of tokens at the beginning of the session. These tokens are not contingent on desirable behaviors. That is, the client does not earn them. During the treatment sessions, you withdraw a token for every undesirable response. You may reinforce the desirable responses with verbal praise and such other social reinforcers that you cannot take back.

In the **earn-and-lose** type of response cost, all tokens are contingent on desirable behaviors. That is, the client must earn them by exhibiting desirable behaviors. While thus earning them, the client loses a token for every instance of an undesirable behavior. In this case, both the desirable and the undesirable behaviors face the token contingency.

Either the lose-only or the earn-and-lose method may be used individually or in small groups. When used with groups, any individual's undesirable behavior will cost the group a token. The group earns tokens only when all members exhibit the desirable behavior.

Like all other response reduction procedures, response cost may be ineffective or may increase the rate of undesirable response under certain conditions. You must carefully avoid the following problems in designing a response cost system for your clients.

1. **Low token loss preceded by high loss may be ineffective.** Typically, you withdraw one token per undesirable response. But in some cases, to make it work, you may have to withdraw multiple tokens per response. If you do this, you should not start with a high number and then go down. For instance, you should not first take away five tokens per undesirable response and then only two. The reduced token loss condition may be ineffective.

2. **The client may run out of tokens.** Then there is nothing to lose and you do not have response cost to reduce the behavior.

3. **Loss of tokens may cause emotional responses.** If such responses do not subside soon, use another method of response reduction. You should not carry the method to a point where you struggle with the client to take tokens away or that the child is in tears.

4. **The undesirable behavior may increase because of attention.** When you take a token away, you also pay immediate, contingent attention to the undesirable response. If the response increases, use another procedure.

How To Use Response Cost. Along with time-out, response cost is a widely researched method of reducing undesirable behaviors. It is known to be very effective, socially acceptable, and less aversive than some of the other methods of behavior reduction. Use the following guidelines in designing a response cost procedure for your client.

1. **Prefer the earn-and-lose method to lose-only method.** This method allows you to systematically reinforce correct and cooperative behaviors through tokens earned while reducing undesirable behaviors through tokens lost.
2. **Give more tokens than you take back.** To this end, simplify the target response and shape it if necessary. The child should experience more success (reinforcers) than failures (token loss). At the end of the session, the child should be left with some tokens that are exchanged for back-up reinforcers.
3. **Withdraw tokens promptly.** There should be no delay between the response and token withdrawal.
4. **If necessary, increase the number of tokens withdrawn per response.** Do this when a single or fewer token withdrawals are not effective. But do not decrease the number of tokens withdrawn.
5. **Avoid client indebtedness.** If you find yourself withdrawing too many tokens resulting in the client debt, switch to another response reduction method.

As with any response reduction procedure, watch for excessive emotional responses and paradoxical increase in undesirable behaviors. Always be ready to use another response reduction procedure.

Extinction. In **extinction,** consequences that reinforce a behavior are withheld. Note that *extinction is not a punishment procedure* while response cost and time-out are. But all three procedures have the same effect on the behavior: reduced frequency. We have grouped extinction along with response cost and time-out to point out that in all three, the locus of contingency management is the undesirable behavior. Though the three procedures are direct compared to procedures that reduce certain behaviors by increasing others, extinction of positively reinforced behaviors is less direct than response cost and time-out. But the extinction of negatively reinforced behavior, as you will find out shortly, is a direct procedure.

In extinction, you do nothing to help sustain the behavior so the behavior is reduced. It is a response-weakening procedure by removing reinforcing consequences. Therefore, you can use this procedure only when the behavior to be reduced is either positively or negatively reinforced. Your functional analysis baselines might suggest that the behavior is indeed maintained by these kinds of reinforcement.

Children's uncooperative behaviors are prime targets for extinction. Such interfering behaviors as crying, fussing, frequent verbal requests to go to the bathroom or see the parent waiting outside, irrelevant talking (the "you know what?" type of interference), and many other similar behaviors are maintained by clinician's reinforcement. The reinforcement may be positive or negative. The clinician may positively reinforce repeated verbal requests to go to the bathroom by paying attention. But leaving the treatment room for the bathroom is a negatively reinforced behavior. The child who leaves the treatment room terminates aversive treatment. This is negative reinforcement. Note that if the child begins to leave the treatment room, you cannot just ignore the behavior. You need to prevent escape, thus depriving the child of negative reinforcement. Prevention of escape is sometimes described as **escape extinction** (Iwata et al., 1990). This procedure implies that extinction is not always a passive or indirect procedure.

How To Use Extinction. In using extinction, follow these guidelines.

1. **Discuss the problem and the extinction procedure with the parents.** Some parents may be alarmed to see you sitting still when their 3-year-old child is loudly and tearfully crying "Mommy!" If they understand what you are doing and why, they may tolerate the procedure. Extinction is slow and unpleasant for both the child and those who administer it or watch it.

2. **Find out what reinforces the undesirable behavior.** Try to find out if the behavior is reinforced positively, negatively, or with a combination of the two. Also, find out if the behavior is reinforced independent of what you do. For example, a child who leaves the chair and goes to the blackboard to scribble may be reinforced independent of your actions. Also, the child is reinforced negatively (escape from your teaching) and positively (scribbling on the blackboard). In this case, even if you avoid all interactions with the child to eliminate reinforcement, the behavior still may persist because of negative and positive reinforcement.

3. **Remove positive reinforcers inherent to your actions promptly and as fully as possible.** Withdraw all attention from the undesirable behavior. Avoid eye contact; sit motionless. Be firm, wait it out; do not change anything. For example, once you initiate extinction for crying behavior, do not lecture; do not admonish; do not cajole; do not try to charm the child; do not try to talk the child out of crying.

4. **Remove positive reinforcers that are unrelated to your actions.** If the child on the floor begins to play with a toy, look

at pictures, examines your bag and so forth, remove the objects promptly and then sit motionless.

5. **Remove negative reinforcers promptly and as fully as possible.** Prevent the child from leaving the seat, walking around or out of the treatment room. Do not stop treatment because the child asks interrupting questions. Do not answer such questions as "Do you know what?" If you answer such questions, you will have positively reinforced such interruptive questioning and negatively reinforced the escape behavior which terminates your teaching.

6. **Do not terminate the extinction procedure when you see an extinction burst.** It is a temporary increase in the rate of a response when extinction is initiated. Continue to withhold reinforcers and the behavior will eventually subside.

7. **Reinforce the desirable behavior promptly and lavishly.** For example, the instant the child stops crying or fussing, smile, hug the child, wipe the tears, praise, give a token, and reinforce the child in other ways. Make the desirable behavior pay off better for the child than the undesirable behavior.

A Word of Caution. Behaviors that are reinforced automatically and those that are destructive or aggressive are not candidates for extinction. You cannot ignore a self-stimulatory behavior and expect it to diminish. Such behaviors are automatically reinforced by their sensory consequences. Aggressive behavior, though facing extinction, might still hurt others. Besides, the behavior itself is not likely to be reduced because of the reinforcement it receives (the effect on others).

Indirect Strategy for Decreasing Behaviors

In the direct strategies of stimulus presentation and stimulus withdrawal (extinction, time-out, and response cost), you place the treatment contingency directly on the undesirable behavior to reduce its frequency. To the contrary, in the **indirect strategy,** you do not place a treatment contingency on the undesirable behavior at all. This approach is so indirect that you do nothing specific to the behavior to be reduced. Instead, you *replace* the undesirable behaviors by desirable behaviors.

The main feature of the indirect strategy is that undesirable behaviors are replaced by certain desirable behaviors which are reinforced. In a sense, you use reinforcement to control undesirable behaviors; by reinforcing desirable behaviors, you weaken undesirable behaviors. But you should never make the mistake of saying that "I use reinforcement to decrease undesirable behaviors." Reinforcement only can increase behaviors. When you use reinforcing procedures, the behavioral reduction is a by-product. Undesirable behaviors decrease only because other behaviors increase. Therefore, you might say that "I use reinforcement to increase some behaviors so that other behaviors are decreased."

The use of reinforcement to increase some behaviors while other behaviors decrease as a result is known as **differential reinforcement**. The term differential suggests that it is not the straightforward reinforcement of some behavior. There is a differential effect of the reinforcement procedure. Although some behaviors increase because of the reinforcement, others decrease as a by-product. This is the meaning of *differential* reinforcement.

There are several differential reinforcement procedures that help you increase some behaviors which would have a concurrent effect of reducing other behaviors. The difference between some of them is subtle and probably not crucial. But if you understand the difference, you will be a sophisticated user of response reduction procedures. The following four differential reinforcement procedures are important: differential reinforcement of other behavior (DRO), differential reinforcement of incompatible behavior (DRI), differential reinforcement of alternative behavior (DRA), and differential reinforcement of low rates of responding (DRL).

Differential Reinforcement of Other Behavior (DRO). In this procedure, you reinforce a child for not exhibiting a specified undesirable behavior for a particular duration. For example, you may reinforce a child for not wiggling in the chair for 2 minutes. If the child omits the behavior for that entire duration, you may give the child a token. Gradually, you can increase the duration for which the child should refrain from the undesirable behavior. A child who frequently interrupts you during treatment may be asked not to do it for a period of several minutes. The child is then reinforced for compliance. An aggressive child may be told that he or she will receive a token if physically or verbally aggressive behavior is not exhibited for a certain duration.

The examples of DRO show that what is reinforced is left open. The procedure does not require a particular desirable behavior to earn reinforcers. The child need not do anything particular to get reinforced; he or she must refrain from doing something (the specified undesirable behavior). An aggressive or hyperactive child, for example, may sit quietly for the specified duration to earn reinforcers. But the child may also read, color, work on math problems, or put puzzles together to earn the reinforcer. You look for these and many other forms of acceptable behaviors, none specified ahead of time, to reinforce. Some desirable behavior and the omission of the specified undesirable behavior results in reinforcement.

Differential Reinforcement of Incompatible Behavior (DRI). In this procedure, you reinforce behaviors that are incompatible with the undesirable behavior. Unlike the DRO in which no specific desirable behavior is required, a behavior that is topographically incompatible with the undesirable behavior is required in DRI and reinforced when it occurs. A child who is verbally abusive may be reinforced for nonabusive, socially acceptable verbal expressions. A child who snatches toys from other children may be reinforced for giving his or her toy to the playmates.

Note that abusive expressions are incompatible with socially acceptable expressions in that both cannot be produced at the same time. Similarly, snatching and sharing do not occur simultaneously. Therefore, when the desirable behavior is increased with reinforcement, the incompatible undesirable behavior should decrease. To use DRI, you must find a response that cannot coexist with the undesirable behavior and target that for reinforcement.

Differential Reinforcement of Alternative Behavior (DRA). In this procedure, you specify and reinforce a behavior that is an alternative to the undesirable behavior. Note that an alternative desirable behavior is not necessarily incompatible with the undesirable behavior to be reduced. In DRA, the desirable behavior is just an alternative to, but not incompatible with, the undesirable behavior. For example, you may find out that a child often is disruptive because of lack of academic or social skills. In this case, you may target specific reading or writing skills and adaptive social skills which the child will enjoy more than the disruptive behaviors.

One drawback with the DRA procedure is that because the desirable behavior is not incompatible with the undesirable behavior, both may be exhibited. While learning better academic and social skills, the child may continue to disrupt. In such cases, it is necessary to teach behaviors that are incompatible with the undesirable behavior.

Differential Reinforcement of Low Rates of Responding (DRL). In this procedure, you reinforce the child when the frequency of undesirable behavior is below the baseline level. In DRL, you shape the undesirable response down until it is eliminated or reduced to a manageable level. The procedure gradually reduces the behavior. For example, you find out that during treatment sessions, a child asks "Are we done yet?" once every 2 to 3 minutes. You can then set a criterion of no more than two interruptions in a 10-minute interval. Normally, the child would have interrupted some three to five times during this interval. You can reinforce the child if during the previous 10-minute duration, the child had interrupted you only two times or less. In using this procedure, you must make sure that you do not reinforce the child soon after an interruption.

Differential reinforcement, especially the DRO, DRI, and the DRA are procedures that help you replace the undesirable behavior with desirable behaviors. In these procedures, while reinforcing desirable behaviors, you make sure that you do not reinforce undesirable behaviors. Therefore, a common theme of these procedures is that (a) the client gains access to reinforcing affairs through desirable behaviors; (b) the undesirable behaviors do not get reinforced anymore; (c) consequently, the undesirable behaviors do not serve the client as they did before; and therefore, (d) the desirable behaviors replace the undesirable behaviors.

General Guidelines for Reducing Undesirable Behaviors

We have described several procedures of response reduction. While each of them may reduce responses, you should not think of using an isolated procedure in reducing or increasing behaviors. You must design a comprehensive program of contingency management involving reinforcement for the desirable responses, withdrawal of reinforcers for the undesirable responses, presentation of response reduction consequences for the undesirable behaviors, and others. A combined procedure that simultaneously shapes and reinforces a desirable behavior while withdrawing reinforcers from the undesirable behaviors and presenting them with other response reduction consequences will be the most effective.

Use the following guidelines in designing an effective response reduction strategy involving multiple contingencies or procedures. Note that the overall strategy includes procedures that increase desirable behaviors. Again, do not confuse the two types of contingencies. You place one kind of contingency on the undesirable behavior and a different kind of contingency on the desirable behavior.

1. **See if response reduction procedures other than extinction may be omitted altogether.** If the undesirable behavior is not frequent enough to disrupt the treatment process, continue to reinforce the desirable behavior and ignore the undesirable behavior. Use one of the response reduction procedures only when this strategy fails to bring the undesirable behavior under a manageable level. For example, if reinforcement of correct articulation is doing the job, ignore the incorrect productions. However, if the incorrect productions persist, introduce a more active response reduction procedure (verbal "No," response cost, or time-out).

2. **Use procedures that help prevent undesirable responses.** Model the correct response until the client's productions stabilize. You then would not have to use the response reduction procedures because the client is successful. Prompt the correct response when the client hesitates; such hesitations may signal an imminent wrong response; you prevent it by prompting the correct response.

3. **Clearly and narrowly define both the undesirable behavior to be reduced and the desirable behavior to be increased.** For instance, "distorted /s/ productions" is a more clearly and narrowly defined response than "problems of articulation." Similarly, "production of part-word repetitions" (and other specific types of dysfluency types) is a more clearly and narrowly defined behavior than "stuttering moment." Conversely, production of correct /s/ is a better definition than "improved articulatory skills." Similarly, "reduced speech rate through syllable prolongation" is a better definition than "controlled rate of speech." Use response reduction procedures only when you have such clearly defined behaviors on which you can place response contingencies.

4. **Differentially reinforce a desirable behavior that is incompatible with the undesirable behavior (DRI).** For instance, in-seat behavior is incompatible with out-of-seat behavior; any form of cooperative behavior does not coexist with noncooperative behavior; attention replaces inattention; smiling and crying are opposite behaviors. To make the response reduction procedure less aversive, reinforce the incompatible desirable response. When you do this, you will simultaneously increase a desirable behavior and decrease an undesirable behavior. This action will help limit the use of aversive response reduction procedures.

5. **Differentially reinforce a desirable behavior that will secure for the client what the undesirable behavior seems to secure (DRA).** Technically, this means that you teach a desirable behavior that is functionally equivalent to the behavior to be reduced (Carr & Durand, 1985). If it looks like the child is crawling under the table to get your attention, then provide lavish attention to quiet sitting in the chair. Children who are minimally verbal or those who are nonverbal may fuss often because that is the only way they can get their wants satisfied. Teaching mands (requests, demands) may reduce such inappropriate behaviors.

6. **Differentially reinforce the client for reducing the rate of the undesirable behavior (DRL).** If you see systematic reduction in the undesirable behavior, reinforce the child while that behavior is not being exhibited. For example, you might tell the child that he wiggled only once during the last 5 minutes and reinforce when sitting without wiggling.

7. **Differentially reinforce the client for simply omitting the undesirable behavior and for producing any of the many acceptable behaviors (DRO).** For example, in a group, reinforce a disruptive child for not being disruptive; your reinforcers may be made contingent on many and unspecified desirable behaviors.

8. **Use varied consequences to reduce a response.** (Charlop, Burgio, Iwata, & Ivancic, 1988). Do not use one type of response consequence constantly. For example, in the same treatment sessions, alternate the use of verbal "No," response cost, time-out, and other consequences that reduce the response rate. Similarly, use varied reinforcers to increase the desirable behavior that will replace the undesirable behavior (Egel, 1981). Verbal praise, tokens backed with many reinforcers, frequent feedback on response accuracy, opportunities for exhibiting high probability behaviors, all may be used in a single sessions.

9. **See if an interfering response may be used to reinforce correct responses** (Charlop, Kurtz, & Kasey, 1990). For example, a child frequently may leave the seat to go to the blackboard and scribble on it. Instead of trying to suppress this interfering behavior with a verbal "No" and such other means, you can make short durations of drawing or writing on the blackboard contingent on sitting for a few minutes and giving correct responses. You will then have turned an

annoying, interfering behavior into a reinforcer of desirable target behaviors.

10. **See if behavioral momentum may be effective in decreasing certain undesirable behaviors.** Behavioral momentum is presumed when the force of a behavior in progress causes another behavior that may not otherwise be exhibited (Mace et al., 1988). In using behavior momentum, you first ask the client to do what he or she is likely to do; as soon as this behavior occurs and it is reinforced, you ask the client to perform an action that he or she is not likely to perform. The unlikely behavior may be performed because of the force (momentum) of the previous, readily exhibited behavior.

    This method has been used to reduce noncompliant behaviors (Mace et al., 1988). For example, assume that a girl does not comply with your request to look at the stimulus picture used in training words. Also assume that she readily will clap her hands when asked to. Then, you could ask her to clap two or three times in succession and immediately ask her to look at the picture. She may then immediately look at the picture. Note that when picture attending behavior increases, the noncompliance behavior will have decreased. You decreased noncompliance behavior by behavior momentum.

11. **See if the undesirable behavior is a means of escape from therapeutic work you demand of the client.** Some children crawl under the table, leave their seat, or look away from you because they find the treatment aversive. By their undesirable behaviors, children escape from therapy or instruction (Carr & Durand, 1985; Iwata, 1987; Iwata et al., 1990). Treatment may be aversive to clients because of many reasons, but the most frequent reason is that the task is too difficult and the child receives too much punishment and too little reinforcement. Then, simplify the task. Shape the target behavior in small steps so that the child is more successful, and hence, receives reinforcement more often.

12. **See if a strong, sudden, and surprising stimulus can terminate or prevent an undesirable behavior.** A study has shown that sudden loud noise can *terminate* undesirable behaviors (Charlop, Burgio, Iwata, & Ivancic, 1988). But you may *prevent* undesirable behaviors by anticipating them and then presenting a sudden and surprising stimulus. For example, a child's imminent crying may be prevented if you suddenly and dramatically pull out a clown or an animated toy

just before the crying is about to erupt. You suddenly may turn on the radio, get up from the chair, pull something from a box or behave in some dramatic fashion. Stimuli that appear so suddenly and dramatically tend to inhibit certain undesirable behaviors.

To prevent undesirable behaviors by sudden stimulus presentation, you must watch the client very closely and observe the early signs of trouble. The stimulus must be presented before the response onset; if not, you may reinforce the undesirable response.

Stimuli that terminate undesirable behaviors are aversives; but those that prevent such behaviors are positive reinforcers. For instance, you say "No" to an undesirable behavior which is promptly terminated. The verbal "No" is an aversive stimulus. To the contrary, when you prevent an imminent crying response by pulling out a clown, you provoke an incompatible response of surprise, curiosity, and so forth. The clown is a positive reinforcer. Be clear about this distinction.

13. **Use a continuous schedule.** Make sure every instance of an undesirable behavior is followed by the response reduction procedure you have selected. Whether it is response cost, time-out, or verbal stimuli, apply it continuously.

14. **Present or withdraw consequences immediately.** Do not hesitate, wait, or be slow in responding to the undesirable response.

15. **Do not allow escape from the response reduction procedure.** A crying child being ignored should not get out of the treatment room only to be consoled by the parent waiting outside. This will positively reinforce the crying behavior. Similarly, clients under other response reduction procedures should not be allowed to leave the treatment scene. If they are, the clients will escape from treatment and get negative reinforcement. (Contrast this with #9; these two are different concepts.)

16. **Apply the response reduction procedure at the earliest sign of the undesirable response.** Do not wait until the undesirable response is completed to apply the procedure. Suppose you wish to reduce a child's behavior of leaving the chair. You should not wait to say "No" until after the child has left the chair and is now on the floor. The best time to say "No" (assuming it will be effective) is when you see the slightest movement of the child that suggests an imminent response. In using time-out for stuttering, you should not wait until an

instance of stuttering has been completed. Instead, you must watch for the earliest signs of stuttering and apply the procedure.

17. **Dissociate response reduction procedures from those that reinforce responses.** You should not deliver reinforcers along with or in close proximity with response reduction procedures. If you do and if it so happens that the reinforcers are stronger than the response reduction procedures, you actually will have reinforced the undesirable behavior. Some clinicians say "Wrong" but immediately smile, touch, or hug the child. These positive responses from the clinician may neutralize the effects of "Wrong" or even reinforce the undesirable response.

18. **Minimize the duration of response reduction procedures.** Time-out should be brief. No response reduction procedure should be applied for too long. If it looks like you have to, you are not using an effective treatment procedure. Maybe you have a wrong or extremely difficult target for the child; maybe you do not have effective reinforcers to increase the desirable behavior; perhaps you are not administering treatment contingencies properly. Analyze your procedures to make them more effective.

19. **Remove reinforcers that maintain undesirable behaviors.** If you see the child constantly reaching for your bag on the table, do not continue to reprimand the child; instead, remove the bag and keep it out of the child's reach and sight. See what reinforces the undesirable behavior. If it is something than can be eliminated, do so immediately.

20. **Make sure the client is exposed to more reinforcing consequences than to response reduction consequences.** Overall, treatment sessions should be much more reinforcing (fun) than aversive to the child. You should be giving more tokens than you withdraw; you should be praising the child more frequently than you reprimand. Of course, to do this, you should be using procedures that help shape the target behaviors.

Aversive Nature of Response Reduction Procedures

Response reduction procedures are aversive not only to clients, but also to clinicians. No clinician enjoys applying aversive procedures. Prudent and limited use of response reduction procedures that are only minimally aversive, socially acceptable, and do not involve emotional or physical harm often are necessary in treatment programs. We have argued that in all treatment sessions, the emphasis should be on positive reinforcement procedures. You should design treatment procedures such that response reduction procedures are avoided; if this is not possible, the need should be minimal.

Always think of simplifying the desirable target response; find an effective reinforcer for it; target alternative, other, or incompatible responses that when increased, will decrease the undesirable behavior. See if extinction will work before you apply more aversive procedures. At the end of the session, count the number of positive reinforcers and response reducing consequences that you delivered. If you have not applied reinforcing consequences more often than the response reduction consequences, critically evaluate your treatment procedures. Discuss this with your clinical supervisor. Remember always, that frequent use of response reduction procedures suggests that something is wrong. Your goal is to avoid response reduction procedures if possible; this requires the most effective way of structuring your treatment program and using the most powerful positive reinforcers.

9

Maintenance of Target Behaviors

You soon will find in your clinical practicum that promoting maintenance of target behaviors in natural settings and over time is a more challenging job than establishing them in the first place. Therefore, you must pay at least as much attention to maintenance strategies as you do to response establishment strategies. In case of persons who stutter, you may have to work harder on fluency maintenance than on establishment.

You often will read that generalization is the final goal of treatment. When a child who learns to produce certain phonemes in the clinic does not pronounce them at home, you are told that the correct production did not generalize. Therefore, you are asked to program generalization before you dismiss the client.

A critical look at generalization shows that it should not be the final goal of treatment. Generalization is a declining rate of response when untrained stimuli are presented and reinforcers are withheld (Hegde, 1985). Generalized but unreinforced responses are extinguished. Therefore, if generalization is the final target, we will have to assume that a declining rate of response is the final goal of treatment. No clinician assumes this. Instead, you are told to have parents and others reinforce generalized responses produced at home and other nonclinical settings. This action leads to a contradictory conclusion that generalized responses are reinforced responses. If so, generalization

227

must be redefined as reinforced responses. There is then no difference between treatment and generalization strategies. Therefore, to avoid all these contradictions, we emphasize that generalization is not the final objective of clinical intervention.

Maintenance of Target Behaviors in Natural Settings

The **final treatment goal is maintenance** of target behaviors. The clinically established communicative behaviors must be produced in conversational speech, in the natural environment, and must be sustained over time. Behaviors that generate favorable consequences are likely to be maintained. If the client reliably produces the behaviors in the clinic but not at home and other settings, then we must have people in those settings do some of the things the clinician did to establish those behaviors. We achieve this by designing a maintenance strategy.

A maintenance strategy is an extension of treatment to natural settings. The main task in implementing a maintenance strategy is to teach people in the life of the client to support and sustain target behaviors. A significant part of the strategy also is to teach the client to manage his or her own behaviors. Therefore, clients, and people who interact with them are the key players in the maintenance strategy.

Maintenance Procedures

To promote maintenance, you must extend treatment to natural settings, but there is nothing substantially new in the maintenance techniques themselves. What is new about the strategy is that the clinician must train others in contingency management at home and at other nonclinical settings.

If treatment is to change the client's behavior, maintenance is used to change the behavior of people around the client. If they continue to behave in their usual manner, the client may not maintain the target responses. Therefore, to implement a maintenance strategy, you should learn to work with parents, spouses, siblings, friends, teachers, and colleagues of the client so that they react differently to the client.

Recall that in Chapter 7, treatment in communicative disorders was defined as a rearrangement of a communicative relationship between the client and his or her listeners. You, the clinician were the initial listener in rearranging that communicative relationship. The final listeners are the people surrounding the client. In both the cases, listeners help change the behavior of the client. While you know how to change the client's (speaker's) behavior, other listeners do not. To help them learn the techniques of changing the behavior of their particular speaker (your client) is the heart of maintenance strategy.

By training the people in the client's life to manage the reinforcement contingencies, you will be shifting the target behavior control from yourself to others. You also will be shifting the location of response control from the clinic to at least a few natural settings. The basic idea here is that like treatment, response maintenance also is a response control procedure.

Besides shifting response control to others, you must take a few other steps as well. Maintenance is a consideration even when you select and teach the target behaviors. As the target behaviors are produced more reliably in the clinical setting, you initiate other, more crucial procedures of response maintenance. Therefore, in a comprehensive maintenance strategy, take the following steps.

Select Useful Behaviors

As pointed out in Chapter 6, behaviors that are useful to the client are more likely to be produced and maintained in natural settings. Communicative behaviors that serve the needs of the client are likely to receive reinforcement from others. Therefore, by selecting client-specific, meaningful, and useful behaviors you set the stage for later maintenance strategy.

Reinforce Target Responses in Conversational Speech

Clinicians sometime fail to move treatment into complex response topography. They may continue for too long at word and phrase levels of training or not spend enough time on training the target behavior in conversational speech. In the natural settings, connected speech is reinforced more readily than words and phrases. Certain other target behaviors, for example fluency and voice qualities, trained only at the word level, may be ineffective when the client speaks continuously in natural settings. Therefore, the target behaviors must always be monitored in conversational speech in the final stages of treatment.

As early as possible, move treatment to conversational speech level. In the treatment of stuttering and voice disorders, move through the simpler levels of words and phrases as rapidly as you can. Spend more clinical time monitoring the target behaviors in conversational speech than in words or phrases. In case of articulation disorders, monitor the correct production of speech sounds in continuous speech. In teaching words to children who are language disordered, move to phrases, sentences, and continuous speech as quickly as possible. Do the same in teaching grammatical morphemes, syntactic structures, and pragmatic features.

Shift Reinforcement Schedules

A behavior reinforced continuously does not resist extinction as much as the one reinforced intermittently. The longer a behavior resists extinction, the greater the chance that it will come under some reinforcement contingency. This situation then will help maintain the target behavior. Therefore, after having established the target behaviors initially through continuous reinforcement, begin to reinforce on an intermittent schedule.

In gradual steps, move from a FR2 to progressively higher ratios. As you decrease the amount of reinforcement, pay close attention to response rates. You may have to lower the ratio if the response rates decline. In the final stages of treatment when the target responses are monitored in conversational speech, reinforce only sporadically.

Use Social and Conditioned Generalized Reinforcers

Social reinforcers are more prevalent in the natural settings. Therefore, even when you have to use primary reinforcers, pair them with social reinforcers, including verbal praise. If the same kinds of reinforcers are encountered in the clinic and natural settings, the responses are more likely to be maintained.

Besides social reinforcers, use conditioned generalized reinforcers. A token system with a variety of back-up reinforcers increases the chances of similar reinforcers being encountered in the natural setting. Also, the family members may be able to implement a similar token system at home to sustain the response rates. The job of the client's family members will be easier if they can use an established system of reinforcement.

Spread the Discriminative Stimulus Control

A discriminative stimulus is a stimulus in whose presence a response has been reinforced. As a result, the response is likely in the presence of that stimulus. Any stimulus may acquire the power to evoke a response because of its systematic association with reinforcement.

The discriminative stimulus will not continue to evoke the response for too long if the response is not reinforced. However, an initial response in the presence of a discriminative stimulus gives the opportunity to reinforce that response to sustain it.

The most important discriminative stimuli are persons, physical stimuli, and physical settings. The clinician is the first discriminative stimulus for the target response. By systematically reinforcing the target response, the clinician comes to exert a strong control over it. Soon, the clinical setting also will come to control the target response.

Some dramatic examples illustrate the power of the clinician and the clinical setting in evoking target responses. For instance, parents often are amazed at the amount of fluency their stuttering children exhibit in front of the clinician and in the treatment room. Anywhere else the children may stutter just as much as they did before treatment. The child who reliably produces words in the treatment room may continue to gesture at home. A woman's hoarseness may all but disappear when she walks into the treatment room. But just as dramatically, her normal sounding voice may disappear as she leaves the clinic. This appearance and disappearance of target behaviors are due to the discriminative stimulus value of the clinician and the treatment room and lack of discriminative stimuli in nonclinical settings.

The task is to spread this discriminative stimulus control exerted almost exclusively by the clinician and the clinical setting to other people and nonclinical settings. When associated with reinforcement, other people and other settings begin to evoke target behaviors. Therefore, to spread the discriminative stimulus value, take the following steps.

Ask the client's family members to sit in the treatment room. If they are associated with treatment and reinforcement, the family members may acquire some power to evoke the target responses at home. Whenever possible, the parents and other members of the family should at least observe the treatment sessions. They should do this not from the other side of one-way mirrors, but by sitting in the treatment room. This is done to associate their presence with treatment. At this stage, family members do not reinforce or do anything else. In the latter stages of treatment, ask your friends or others who are strangers to the client to observe treatment sessions. Make sure you discuss this with parents and clients before you invite other persons to sessions because it raises the issue of confidentiality. You need the permission of adult clients and parents or guardians of minors.

Move treatment to outside the treatment room. The restricted treatment room is useful and often necessary to establish target behaviors because it provides a controlled environment free of distraction. But the room is so different from the client's everyday environment that the client's learning is restricted to its confines. Therefore, when the client begins to produce the target behaviors in conversational speech, move treatment out of the treatment room. Take a walk with the client outside the clinic. Converse with the client and monitor the production of target behaviors in conversational speech.

If the client's response rates drop dramatically when you move out of the treatment room, and you find it hard to control this drop, move back into the treatment room and try again sometime later. If the client sustains the responses, then move to progressively more different situations. Take the client to shopping centers, restaurants, bookstores, toy stores, and other relevant places and have the client talk to people there. Use the following guidelines in carrying out this procedure.

1. **In the beginning, take the client to less threatening situations.** You may not even ask the client to talk to any strangers the first time you two go outside the clinic. Let the client talk to you in the new environment while you monitor and reinforce the target responses.
2. **Let the client rehearse what he or she will tell a stranger in a new setting.** For example, you might have a stuttering client talk to a bookstore clerk. What the client plans to tell the clerk should be rehearsed with your help so that he or she can speak slowly and fluently.
3. **The first few times, stay close to the client.** If needed, give a subtle signal to trigger the target response. You may touch the client's shoulder as he or she begins to speak to prompt the correct response. In the case of a stuttering man, for example, the touch may mean that he must slow down his rate.
4. **Take note of the correct and incorrect productions.** Give subtle and quick reinforcement. This is important because the strangers the clients talk to will not reinforce. It is your reinforcement in these new situations that will establish the discriminative stimulus value of those situations and listeners.

5. **Gradually increase the distance between you and your client.** As the client begins to talk to strangers, slowly move away from them.
6. **Take the client to progressively more difficult situations.** As the target responses are maintained in each new situation, take the client to a more difficult situation. Reinforce the client in all situations.

Teach Others To Evoke and Consequate Target Behaviors

This technique is the heart of maintenance strategy; it can and must be implemented whether there is initial generalization or not. Treatment will have been extended to the natural environment if the significant others in the client's life know (a) the exact target behaviors, (b) how to evoke them, and (c) how to consequate them. The target behaviors then have the greatest probability of being maintained.

Take the following steps in teaching others to evoke and consequate target behaviors.

1. **Describe and demonstrate the target behaviors to others.** When you invite the family members and others to observe the treatment sessions, describe the target behaviors being taught. Tell them precisely what the client is expected to do. Do not use jargon. Give simple and direct descriptions. For example, while treating a child who stutters, say "I want Johnny to talk very slowly. Perhaps as slowly as I am talking now. [Model the target rate.] Johnny should stretch his words like this. [Model a few words by prolonging the syllables.] When Johnny stretches his words, he does not stutter that much. When he practices slower speech without stuttering for a while, he can begin to speak a little faster until his speech will sound OK and he will be speaking more fluently."

   While teaching a set of basic words to a child who is language delayed, tell the parents you are teaching a few words, not a "core vocabulary." When you have to use technical terms (e. g., present progressive or prepositions), give examples. Show the parents and other members of the family a list of words, phrases, and sentences you teach the child.

   In treating voice disorders, contrast the desirable and undesirable voice or resonance qualities. In simple terms, describe the relation between vocal abuse and voice problems. With the help of charts and drawings, show them how the vocal mechanism works and how important it is to maintain appropriate vocal behaviors.

2. **Demonstrate how to evoke target behaviors.** Let family members watch you evoke the target behaviors. They should know how to model the target behaviors for the client. Although they are not expected to shape the behavior or model excessively at home, the parents, spouses, and siblings should suggest the target behavior when the client fails to produce it at home. For instance, the members of a stuttering person's family should model the correct way of slowing the rate of speech. They should do it by stretching the words, and not by giving gaps between words. The family members of a child with a language delay or articulation problem should know how to quickly and correctly model words, phrases, and sentences under training.

When the parents begin their work at home, the need to model extensively will not be crucial. You will have established the target behaviors. Most likely, the parents will have to prompt the target responses. When prompts do not work, the parents must stop the client, remind the target behavior, and perhaps model as well.

Teach parents the subtle ways of prompting the target behavior. When family members begin to modify the client's behavior in natural settings, loud and obvious signals are not acceptable to clients. Especially when prompts have to be given in the presence of guests and visitors, the prompts must be so subtle that the others present do not notice them. A subtle and brief hand gesture or even a movement of a finger may be all that is needed to slow down the rate of speech, reduce the vocal pitch, increase vocal intensity, and decrease hoarseness of voice. Similar gestures can be devised to remind the client to open his or her mouth to increase oral resonance or to assume a certain articulatory posture. A person sitting next to the client at the dining table may touch the client to use a target response. For each specific target response, you must devise such a specific, brief signal.

You should demonstrate selected unobtrusive signals and teach the client to respond reliably to them in the clinic. Then ask the parents to give those signals frequently at home. Some clients may need a more pronounced stimulus in the beginning. If so, in progressive steps, reduce that obvious stimulus to a brief signal that only the family and the client will know has transpired.

During treatment sessions, give the same signal you ask the family members to use at home. When you take the client out of the treatment room to natural settings, experiment with different types of signals, and find out which one works the best for the client. Ask the parents to use the same signal at home.

Family members and others also should be trained to give opportunities for the client to produce the target behaviors. Often, clients who are communicatively handicapped are reluctant to talk even when their problems have been mostly remediated. Persons who stutter or those with hearing loss may talk less in groups as they did before, though they are now expected to use their newly acquired skills of fluency or oral language. Treated persons with aphasia also may be reluctant to talk in front of other persons. A child who has just learned to say some words may not speak them. Having gotten used to their role as silent partners, the family and friends may not ask the person who is communicatively handicapped to take part in conversation. The family and other persons should be trained to expect newly acquired behaviors from the client and give the client sufficient opportunities to express himself or herself.

3. **Teach how to consequate target behaviors.** The client's family, teachers, friends, or colleagues should know how to reinforce the target behavior productions at home and in other situations. Point out to parents and others the importance of reinforcing immediately and demonstrate how to do it. Also, tell them it is equally important to stop the client at the earliest sign of a wrong response. Ask them not to wait until a lengthy but wrong response is completed. Show how you do it.

Like prompts that help evoke the responses in natural settings, response consequences also should be delivered in a subtle manner. Most clients do not want to be reinforced in front of other persons. A man who stutters does not want his wife to say "You are very fluent honey!" in front of formal dinner guests. But reinforcing a stuttering person for speaking fluently in such formal occasions is important. Therefore, a special signal that is not a prompt, but a reinforcement may be given discretely. If such signals are used often in the company of strangers and acquaintances, and backed-up by verbal praise as soon as possible, the signals may act as discriminative stimuli.

Generally, parents and others should be trained to reinforce more often than to punish. When wrong responses are produced, it is better to give a swift prompt than to give a punishing signal. For example, it is better to prompt a stuttering person who starts with a fast rate to slow down the rate than to whisper "No!" A hand gesture to slow down is more neutral than such verbal punishers, and may be more effective. Therefore, train family members and others to reinforce correct responses and prompt correct responses when incorrect responses seem imminent.

Some incorrect responses may continue to be reinforced by the family members. For example, the previously nonverbal child may continue to get reinforced for gestures at home. When it is clear that the child can use words, parents and others should withhold reinforcers for gestures and other nonverbal behaviors. They should immediately prompt correct responses and reinforce them promptly.

Parents and others need not reinforce continuously. By the time the maintenance strategies are begun at home, the client will have been reinforced in the clinic on a fairly large intermittent schedule. Therefore, infrequent reinforcement might be effective. Ask family members to increase the frequency of reinforcement only when the correct responses do not seem to be nearly as high as they are in treatment sessions.

In some cases, when parents, siblings, spouses, teachers, colleagues, and others are able to give an occasional prompt and reinforcement for correct responses, maintenance may be enhanced. In other cases, more extensive and frequent monitoring of the client responses may be needed. How the clients and their family members perform their respective tasks will tell you how much to train and with what degree of precision.

To assess whether family members and others are prompting and reinforcing the target behaviors as expected, you should ask them to tape record a sample conversation or other kinds of exchange and bring it to you. You should ask for such tape recorded evidence periodically to give them feedback on the performance of the family members. If they are making mistakes, you should catch them as soon as possible and give them corrective instructions.

Though most often you train parents to promote maintenance of target behaviors, you may sometimes train them to conduct treatment at home. For example, while working with small children and infants, you often have to train parents to conduct some portion of treatment at home. Infant language stimulation, early intervention for stuttering and articulation disorders, and intervention for vocal abuse in young children may require a substantial amount of parental work. How to train parents to do this is discussed in a subsequent section on developing home management programs.

If parents and spouses can be trained to hold brief and parallel training sessions at home, responses may be stabilized at home sooner than otherwise expected. Possibly, parents and spouses who are also therapists in an informal or limited sense will better promote response maintenance. If parents and spouses cannot do this, at least a few minutes of brief informal sessions at home are highly desirable. When family members agree to do this, they should set aside a time for speech work at home. They should tape record each session they hold and submit it to you for your feedback.

Training significant persons in a client's life is perhaps the most challenging and yet the most necessary task in promoting maintenance. You will have to constantly think of new ways of meeting this challenge.

Teach the Client Self-Control

Self-control is not a mentalistic notion. It is a teachable behavior. We try to control our behaviors with varying degrees of success. But clients who learn to systematically control their behaviors have constant therapists in themselves. Clients who can monitor their behaviors do not depend much on family and friends to sustain their communicative behaviors. Therefore, teaching self-control is an important task in promoting response maintenance.

From the beginning, ask clients to judge the accuracy of their behaviors. Ask the child in articulation treatment to say whether his or her productions were correct or not. In a matter of few training trials, most children can make this judgment. Children who are encouraged to make those judgments frequently begin to monitor their behaviors more closely. They stop as soon as they begin to misarticulate a sound.

A person getting treatment for stuttering may be asked to judge the occurrence of stutterings, abrupt onset of phonation, faster than the required rate of speech, muscular tension while speaking, and most other target responses. Likewise, they can judge the occurrence of smooth phonation, desired rate, relaxed articulation, and so forth. Stuttering speakers who appreciate the contrast between their stuttered speech and the target fluency skills will begin to monitor their speech production. They are likely to stop at the very beginning of a stutter. With further training in self-monitoring, they may stop as soon as they feel tension in their speech musculature and start with greater relaxation. When clients use such tactics, the clinician can reduce the amount of response consequation.

Clients who become more proficient in recognizing their own correct and incorrect responses may be asked to chart their behaviors along with you. Ask them to make a tally mark on a sheet of paper every time they stutter, articulate a phoneme incorrectly, produce an undesirable vocal characteristic, and so forth. Also, ask them to tally their correct responses. Many children are eager to do it. Other children may be asked to count their correct and incorrect behaviors by placing different colored plastic chips in two cups placed in front of them.

Once your clients are able to measure their correct and incorrect behaviors in the clinic, you should ask them to bring data on their performance outside the clinic. Measuring their behaviors in outside situations will help them monitor their target responses more closely. Stuttering individuals may be asked to record the frequency of their dysfluencies in situations where tape recording their speech is not practical. Adult voice clients also may record the frequency of occurrence of hoarseness or hard glottal attacks and so forth. Small, hand-held counters may be used to record the frequency of behaviors.

Another useful strategy of self-control for many clients is to implant signals that remind them of the target behaviors in their everyday situations. For instance, stuttering and high-pitched voice clients may draw arrows pointing downward on small pieces of paper and paste them on telephone receivers, office desks, and other places where they need reminders to reduce the rate of speech or the pitch of their voice.

Clients also may be trained to consequate their own behaviors. Self-administered consequences can be more immediate than those administered by the clinician. A voice or a fluency client may feel subtle tension in the throat that is a signal for stuttering or hoarseness. The clinician may not be able to consequate this without using a biofeedback unit. But if the client can be trained to pause, relax, and try again, such subtle muscular signals of impending incorrect behaviors will be modified before they occur. This is excellent self-control. Some clients may be trained to self-administer time-out. A man who stutters, for example, may be trained to stop speaking for a few seconds each time he stutters. By doing this, he may be able to reduce his stutterings even when no one is monitoring his fluency and stuttering.

Teach the Client To Prime Others To Consequate

A common problem with contingency management in everyday life is that people punish each other more often than they reinforce. When a person does something bad, everyone seems to notice it right away. But when the same person does something good, people are too busy to notice.

Family members and others who are asked to help the client may do the same thing. They may not notice the production of correct behaviors, or take them for granted. They may think that their only job is to stop undesirable behaviors. They may not realize that it is more important to encourage the desirable behavior. For instance, parents who are asked to monitor their child's correct and incorrect productions of target phonemes may notice incorrect production more often than correct productions. The child then hears more critical words than encouraging words.

To counter this tendency, you will have impressed upon the family the need to prompt and reinforce as often as they can and punish as minimally as they have to. Still, many people in the client's life may be slow to reinforce. Therefore, you should teach clients to prime others to reinforce them. **Priming** is a special way of prompting others to reinforce; it is done by those who wish to receive reinforcement. The clinician asks the parent to reinforce their daughter for her correct production of phonemes. At home, the daughter primes her parents to reinforce her correct productions.

Reinforcement priming is done by drawing other people's attention to one's own behaviors that are expected to be reinforced. Whenever we show off our good behaviors or point out something we did well, we may be priming for reinforcement. We may do it with people who are notorious for ignoring good behaviors in others.

Teach clients to draw attention to their target behavior productions and ask the family members to reinforce immediately. Tell the family that you want the client to draw attention. Otherwise, they may think the client is showing off. A girl may point out to her parents that she correctly produced the phoneme throughout a segment of conversation. A stuttering man may remind his wife that he has been speaking fluently for several minutes. Or, soon after fluently ordering food in a restaurant, he may draw his wife's attention to his successful but previously troubled performance. A woman with hoarseness may tell her listeners that she has been speaking very softly or very little in an otherwise loud family discussion.

Vocal emphasis on a target language feature may be another way of drawing attention to it. A boy who has learned to produce the regular plural morpheme slightly emphasizes it in his words, phrases, and sentences. This vocal emphasis may draw the ignoring parent's attention.

You may train clients to ask their friends and family to remind them with a subtle hint that an undesirable response has been made. A woman with pitch breaks may request her roommate to signal with her finger that pitch breaks occurred. A stuttering woman may ask her husband to stop her whenever she stutters or speaks rapidly.

Give Sufficient Treatment

A simple reason why many clients do not maintain target responses is that they have terminated treatment against your advice or you have dismissed the client from services prematurely. There is not much you can do when clients discontinue therapy for reasons unrelated to your effectiveness. The family may move out of the area or run out of resources to continue treatment. But if the treatment was discontinued because they did not see much progress, you have something to think about. You must change or improve your treatment procedures. This is not an issue of maintenance, as the treatment was not completed. It is a maintenance issue when you prematurely dismiss a client who has been showing good progress.

Clients may be prematurely dismissed because the target responses are produced reliably in the clinical setting. The clinician may not realize that much work still needs to be done. For example, a child who correctly produces phonemes in words may still need help in producing them in conversational speech. A man who has learned to maintain an appropriate vocal pitch in the clinic may still be speaking with his unacceptably high pitch elsewhere. A woman with aphasia may be saying a few words in the clinic, but cannot remember any of them after the treatment sessions. But in all such cases, the clinician may dismiss the client from services because the target behaviors are produced at some level of response topography in the clinical setting.

When clients are prematurely dismissed, either the target responses have not been trained sufficiently in conversational speech or no maintenance procedures have been implemented. Because maintenance is treatment also, prematurely dismissed clients will not have received sufficient treatment. More importantly, treatment may be insufficient regardless of maintenance procedures. In this case, treatment will not have sufficiently strengthened the target behaviors. Also, maintenance procedures may have been started prematurely. Some clients who make rapid progress in treatment may show shaky but quick generalization, creating an illusion that sufficient treatment was given. Therefore, the clinician must strengthen complex response topographies in the clinic by intermittent reinforcement. Then the treatment should be gradually extended to natural settings.

Give Booster Treatment

Some clinicians assert that treatment is not successful unless clients are "permanently cured" so that they never need our services for the rest of their lives. Any relapse of stuttering in a treated person often is sharply pointed out by critics who claim there is no successful treatment for stuttering. Voice disorders too, tend to relapse in some cases, and the same argument is made. But a successfully treated disorder may return and this is not necessarily a negative reflection on the previous success. No medical disease, when cured, comes with a guarantee that the patient will not catch the same disease again. Similarly, successful treatment of stuttering or any other communicative disorder does not come with a guarantee that clients will be free from the disorder for the rest of their lives.

Communicative disorders that return after successful treatment suggest that the conditions that create the disorder were confronted again by the person who was treated. We may not fully understand these conditions, or if we did, we may have no control over them. This is a matter for further research.

Meanwhile, the clinician can take pride when a disorder is treated successfully though the likelihood of relapse is there. But a careful clinician plans to take care of this eventuality. Therefore, tell your clients, especially the fluency and voice clients, that they may need additional treatment sometime in the future. Assure them that when the problem emerges again, it can be handled successfully. Caution them though, that they should contact you at the earliest sign of relapse. A slight increase in dysfluencies, hoarseness or harshness of voice, undesirable pitch, and so forth must be brought to the clinician's attention. The sooner the process of relapse is caught, the faster the progress in resumed treatment.

Treatment resumed for a client sometime after dismissal is called **booster treatment**. The need for booster treatment shows that we have many problems to solve in the maintenance of treatment gains. But until research solves them, we must have a schedule for booster treatment for every client who needs it.

The need for booster treatment is most acute for stuttering persons. Most if not all successfully treated stuttering children and adults need booster treatment sometime after they were dismissed from the original treatment. Fluency is not maintained in many treated individuals not because the original therapy was useless, but because they did not receive booster treatment. Therefore, plan on giving booster treatment to every person treated for stuttering.

Booster treatment is typically the same treatment that was successful before unless something more powerful has been developed since then. However, technical improvements made during the intervening time should be included in booster treatment.

The duration of booster treatment is typically brief. In most cases, a few sessions may be sufficient, especially if the client has come back in the early stage of relapse. If the relapse is substantial, booster treatment may be prolonged.

Some clients need repeated booster treatments spread over a few years. Though discouraging to most clients, if it is explained to them that a few repetitions of treatment is a method of fading the treatment out completely, the clinician is likely to have their cooperation.

Booster treatment is also an opportunity to strengthen the family members' skills in monitoring the client's target behaviors. It is possible that as the client's target behaviors deteriorated, the family members' monitoring of those behaviors also deteriorated. More importantly, the target behaviors may have been lost because of the deterioration in the monitoring skills of family members.

Booster treatment is interlinked with follow-up assessments discussed in the final section of this chapter. Extension of treatment to the natural environment coupled with a schedule of follow-up and booster treatment are the best the current treatment technology can offer to maintain target behaviors across speaking situations and over time.

Developing Home Treatment Programs

Home treatment programs are different from maintenance programs implemented by families. When families implement a home maintenance program, they deal with behaviors already established by a clinician. In implementing a home treatment program, the parents may have to establish at least some of the behaviors. The primary treatment responsibility normally rests with the clinician but in home treatment programs, that responsibility is assigned to family members.

Home treatment programs especially are recommended for infants at risk for developing communicative disorders. Among others, infants who show early signs of mental retardation, potential hearing problems, neurological impairment, language delay, or certain genetic syndromes are candidates for early intervention. Early intervention by professionals may not be practical because of lack of trained personnel, clinical facilities, and funds to pay for extended professional help. In such cases, parent training in early intervention may be the only practical course.

Home treatment programs also are needed in cases where clients receive limited treatment from professionals with the understanding that the family members will continue some systematic treatment at home. Clients and families who go out of town to consult with a speech-language pathologist who specializes in the treatment of certain disorders are in this category. In such cases, clients of any age may receive home treatment from their family.

Developing home treatment programs requires more information than can be offered here. You must consult other sources for details (McDonald, 1978; McDonald & Gillette, 1986; Odom & Karnes, 1988; Rossetti, 1986; Tjossem, 1976). Only a few basic principles of developing a home training program are summarized in this section.

Home training programs must be recommended only after the clinician (a) has made a thorough assessment of the client; (b) has developed and tried an intervention program that works; (c) has trained the parents in the home treatment program including objective record keeping procedures; and (d) can make himself or herself available to supervise the family members' work, assess the data supplied by them, modify the treatment program, and retrain the family members when necessary. The clinician should never simply give a written home program and ask them to follow it.

A thorough **assessment** of the infant or the child should include an evaluation of communicative behaviors or their potential. In the case of infants, the early signs of speech and language are assessed. Such behaviors as attention, social smile, play, social or emotional responses to other people, interaction with other children, general motor development, physical development, babbling and cooing, early speech sound productions, single word productions, use of words in social communication, are among the several aspects of child development that are assessed. Besides, sensory development, intellectual status, neurological and physical health of the infant also are assessed by psychologists and medical specialists. Unless a team of specialists have made a complete assessment of the child or infant, it may not be appropriate to recommend an extensive home communication treatment program. Most likely, children who need home treatment programs have other disabilities for which different specialists also will develop home treatment programs. For example, programs for motor, sensory, and physical development may be recommended.

The speech-language pathologist must **develop and experiment** with a treatment program with the infant or the child to make sure it works. Because what works with one infant may not necessarily work with another, the clinician must use a trial period of treatment to establish effective target behaviors and treatment procedures. A few days or weeks of systematic work by the clinician is necessary before a program may be recommended for home use. Continuous data recorded during treatment should be used to assess the infant learning under treatment.

The trial treatment is also the opportunity to **train the parents** in the home treatment program. Parents should take part in all sessions of trial therapy. They should also take part in the selection of target behaviors and in further refining them as treatment continues. They should know how to move on to more complex targets. By initially watching how the clinician uses the procedures, and then implementing those procedures in the presence of the clinician, the parent learns to teach communicative behaviors. During the trial treatment, the clinician should teach the parent the methods of recording the child's responses and in general record keeping procedures.

Assessment of treatment data and **periodic supervision** of parents' work at home is essential to avoid mistakes in implementation. Tape recorded samples of treatment sessions, and preferably, video taped samples, must be evaluated by the clinician. The clinician should promptly review parents' charts and recording sheets to evaluate changes in the infant's behavior. Frequent telephone contact may be necessary to answer their questions and offer suggestions based on submitted data. Periodically, the clinician may visit the home and observe the parents. At this time, the clinician may demonstrate new procedures.

When the data show no significant progress under a home treatment program, formal treatment by a speech-language pathologist must be started. This may have to be done regardless of home progress if the communicative handicaps warrant systematic, formal, professional help.

Follow-Up Assessments

Follow-up is an assessment of response maintenance over time. It is a conversational probe of communicative behaviors. Students in clinical practicum often do not work long enough with the same clients to make follow-up assessments. Each semester of clinical practice, you may be assigned different clients. But follow-up is an important part of clinical work. Even if you did not have frequent opportunities to practice follow-up assessments, you must know the procedures. You will be making those assessments when you take a professional position.

An individualized follow-up schedule is prepared before the client is dismissed from treatment. How the client has progressed often dictates how soon and how often follow-ups are scheduled. Due to practical reasons, a client may be dismissed sooner than expected with the understanding that the client will return for an assessment sooner than usual. A strong response rate at a very high level of accuracy maintained in natural settings on repeated measures may suggest that the first follow-up need not be too soon.

Typically, the first follow-up assessment is scheduled 3 months after the client is dismissed from services. Assuming that the client has maintained the communicative behaviors, the next assessment may be scheduled after 6 months. If the behaviors are maintained, subsequent assessments may be scheduled in yearly intervals. A 3- to 4-year follow-up is needed for speakers who received treatment for their stuttering. A similar schedule may be needed for voice clients. Children who have received treatment for articulation disorders probably do not need to be followed up that long. If correct production of articulation is maintained for a year or so, chances of misarticulations returning may not be great. With other clients, such as those with aphasia or progressive neurological and physical diseases, follow-up assessment schedule is based on the client's health and progress in speech or language treatment.

Timely follow-up assessments help determine the need for booster treatment. These assessments must be used to prevent significant deterioration in target behaviors by offering booster treatment at the earliest possible time. Therefore, in a typical follow-up, take a conversational speech sample. Make this an extended sample. Make it as naturalistic as possible. If time permits, record the sample in a nonclinical setting as well. Take the client out for a walk and engage in conversation. Use a micro tape recorder to record the conversation. Give a test only if it samples connected speech and it gives you some unique data.

Because such tests are practically nonexistent, an extended conversational speech is your best measure.

In sampling language features, you may have to contrive the conversation or direct it in some specific manner to have the client produce those features. Follow the guidelines given in Appendix F on taking conversational speech samples.

Calculate the percent correct response rate for the speech or language sample. Analyze the sample to derive such quantitative data as the following.

- Percentage of dysfluency rate
- Percentage of correct production of phonemes
- Percentage correct use of grammatical morphemes and other language features
- The number of words in sentences
- Percentage of speech time a particular voice quality was maintained
- Frequency of pitch breaks per minute of continuous speech
- Percentage of words on which inappropriate nasal resonance was heard
- Percentage of spoken words that were intelligible
- The number of words or syllables spoken per minute

If the follow-up assessment data suggest that the target behaviors are not maintained or have declined in frequency, arrange for immediate booster treatment. Remember, the goal of follow-up is to assess response maintenance and to give timely booster treatment to those who need it.

Though you have a follow-up schedule, the client and the family must be told they should contact you for an assessment or consultation as soon as they notice a response deterioration. If they do not understand this, the clients and the family may wait for a scheduled follow-up to seek booster treatment. A follow-up schedule is valid only when target behaviors do not deteriorate in the meanwhile.

Much clinical research needs to be done on maintenance of clinically established target behaviors in natural settings. If you approach the problem from the standpoint of extending treatment to nonclinical settings, you may experience greater success than if you tried to "program generalization." Scheduled follow-up and booster treatment and further training of the family members in contingency management during booster sessions are additional features of a sound maintenance strategy.

References

ASHA Committee on Language, Speech, & Hearing Services in the Schools. (1984). Guidelines for caseload size for speech-language services in the schools. *Asha, 26,* 53-57.

ASHA Committee on Quality Assurance. (1989). AIDS/HIV: Implications for speech-language pathologists & audiologists. *Asha, 31,* 33.

ASHA Committee on Quality Assurance. (1990). Update. AIDS/HIV: Implications for speech-language pathologists & audiologists. *Asha, 32,* 46-48.

ASHA Committee on Supervision. (1985). Clinical supervision in speech-language pathology. *Asha, 27,* 57-60.

ASHA Congressional Relations Division, Government Affairs Department. (1989). *Current federal legislative regulatory issues: Issues of interest to speech-language pathologists and persons with communication disorders.* Rockville, MD: American Speech-Language-Hearing Association.

ASHA Council on Professional Ethics. (1991). Code of ethics of the American Speech-Language-Hearing Association, 1991. *Asha, 33,* 103-104.

ASHA Council on Professional Ethics. (1991). Proposed revision of the code of ethics, American Speech-Language-Hearing Association. *Asha, 33,* 65-66.

ASHA Council on Professional Standards in Speech-Language Pathology and Audiology. (1990). Standards for accreditation of educational programs. *Asha, 32,* 93-100.

ASHA Council on Professional Standards in Speech-Language Pathology and Audiology. (1991). Standards for the certificate of clinical competence. *Asha, 33,* 121-122.

ASHA Council on Professional Standards. (1991). Revision of certification standard 111B, clinical practicum, CCC-A. *Asha, 33,* 65.

ASHA Governmental Affairs Review. (1990). *Reauthorization of EHA discretionary programs.* Rockville, MD: American Speech-Language-Hearing Association.

ASHA Membership and Certification Handbook. (1990). Rockville, MD: American Speech-Language-Hearing Association.

ASHA Professional Services Board. (1984). Organization and maintenance of records for clinical service delivery. *Asha, 26,* 39.

Benenson, A.S. (1990). *Control of communicable diseases in man* (15th ed.). Washington DC.: American Public Health Association.

Bernthal, J. E., & Bankson, N. W. (1988). *Articulation and phonological disorders.* Englewood Cliffs, NJ: Prentice-Hall.

Bloodstein, O. (1987). *A handbook on stuttering.* Chicago: National Easter Seal Society.

Boone, D. R. (1972). *Cerebral palsy.* New York: Bobbs-Merrill.

Boone, D. R., & McFarlane, S. C. (1988). *The voice and voice therapy.* (4th ed.). Englewood Cliffs, NJ: Prentice-Hall.

California State Department of Education. (1989). *Program guidelines for language, speech, & hearing specialists providing designated instruction and services.* Sacramento, CA: Author.

Carr, E., & Durand, V. M. (1985). Reducing behavioral problems through functional communication training. *Journal of Applied Behavior Analysis, 18,* 111-126.

Charlop, M. H., Burgio, L. D., Iwata, B. A., & Ivancic, M. T. (1988). Stimulus variation as a means of enhancing punishment effects. *Journal of Applied Behavior Analysis, 21,* 89-95.

Charlop, M. H., Kurtz, P. F., & Casey, F. G. (1990). Using aberrant behaviors as reinforcers for autistic children. *Journal of Applied Behavior Analysis, 23,* 163-181.

Chomsky, N., & Halle, M. (1968). *The sound pattern of English.* New York: Harper & Row.

Darley, F.L., & Spriestersbach, D.C. (1978). *Diagnostic methods in speech pathology* (2nd ed.). New York, NY: Harper & Row.

Davis, G. A. (1983). *A survey of adult aphasia.* Englewood Cliffs, NJ: Prentice-Hall.

Dublinske, S., & Healey, W.C. (1978). P.L. 94-142: Questions and answers for the speech-language pathologist and audiologist. *Asha, 20,* 188-205.

Durand, V. M., & Carr, E. G. (1987). Social influences on "self-stimulatory" behavior: Analysis and treatment application. *Journal of Applied Behavior Analysis, 20,* 119-132.

Egel, A. L. (1981). Reinforcer variation: Implications for motivating developmentally disabled children. *Journal of Applied Behavior Analysis, 14,* 345-350.

Elbert, M., & Gierut, J. (1986). *Handbook of clinical phonology.* Austin, TX: PRO-ED.

Emerick, L.L., & Haynes, W.O. (1986). *Diagnosis and evaluation in speech pathology.* (3rd ed.). Englewood Cliffs, NJ: Prentice-Hall.

Flower, R. (1984). *Delivery of speech-language pathology and audiology services.* Baltimore, MD: Williams & Wilkins.

Hegde, M. N. (1985). *Treatment procedures in communicative disorders.* Austin, TX: PRO-ED.

Hegde, M. N. (1988). *Principles of management and remediation.* In N. J. Lass, L. V. McReynolds, J. L. Northern, & D. F. Yoder (Eds.), Handbook of speech-language pathology & audiology (pp. 377-394). Toronto, Canada: Decker

Hodson, B. W. (1980). *The assessment of phonological processes.* Austin, TX: PRO-ED.

Ingham, R. J. (1984). *Stuttering and behavior therapy: Current status and experimental foundations.* Austin, TX: PRO-ED.

Iwata, B. (1987). Negative reinforcement in applied behavior analysis: An emerging technology. *Journal of Applied Behavior Analysis, 20,* 361-378.

Iwata, B. A., Pace, G. M., Kalsher, M. J., Cowdery, G. E., & Cataldo, M. F. (1990). Experimental analysis and extinction of self-injurious escape behavior. *Journal of Applied Behavior Analysis, 23,* 11-27.

James, S. L. (1990). *Normal language acquisition.* Boston: Little, Brown.

Johns, D. F. (1985). *Clinical management of neurogenic communicative disorders.* Austin, TX: PRO-ED.

Knepflar, K. J., & May, A. A. (1989). *Report writing in the field of communication disorders: A handbook for students & clinicians* (2nd ed.). Rockville, MD: National Student Speech-Language-Hearing Association.

Lynch, C. (1990). Characteristics of state licensure laws. *Asha, 32,* 47-55.

Mace, C. F., Hock, M., Lalli, J. S., West, B. J., Belfiore, P., Pinter, E., & Brown, D. K. (1988). Behavioral momentum in the treatment of noncompliance. *Journal of Applied Behavior Analysis, 21,* 123-141.

Mason, S. A., & Iwata, B. A. (1990). Artifactual effects of sensory-integrative therapy on self-injurious behaviors. *Journal of Applied Behavior Analysis, 23,* 361-370.

McCormick, L., & Schiefelbusch, R. L. (1990). *Early language intervention: An introduction* (2nd ed.). Columbus, OH: Merrill.

McDonald, J. (1978). *Environmental language inventory.* Columbus, OH: Merrill.

McDonald, J., & Gillette, Y. (1986). Communicating with persons with severe handicaps: Roles of parents and professionals. *Journal of the Association for the Severely Handicapped, 11,* 225-265.

McMillan, M.O., & Willette, S.J. (1988). Aseptic technique: A procedure for preventing disease transmission in the practice environment. *Asha, 30,* 35-37.

Musselwhite, C. R., & St. Louis, K. W. (1988). *Communication programming for persons with severe handicaps.* Austin, TX: PRO-ED.

Odom, S., & Karnes, M. (1988). *Early intervention for infants and children with handicaps.* Baltimore: Paul H. Brookes.

Owens, R. E., Jr. (1988). *Language development: An introduction.* Columbus, OH: Merrill.

Owens, R. E., Jr. (1991). *Language disorders: A functional approach to assessment and intervention.* New York: Macmillan.

Peterson, H., & Marquardt, T. (1990). *Appraisal and diagnosis of speech and language disorders* (2nd ed.). Englewood Cliffs,NJ: Prentice-Hall.

Reed, V. A. (1986). *An introduction to children with language disorders.* New York: Macmillan.

Repp, A, C., Felce, D., & Barton, L. E. (1988). Basing the treatment of stereotypic and self-injurious behaviors on hypotheses of their causes. *Journal of Applied Behavior Analysis, 21,* 281-289.

Rosenbek, J. C. (1985). Treating apraxia of speech. In D. F. Johns (Ed.), *Clinical management of communicative disorders* (2nd ed., pp. 276-312). Austin, TX: PRO-ED.

Rosenbek, J. C., LaPointe, L. L., & Wertz, R. (1989). *Aphasia: A clinical approach.* Austin, TX: PRO-ED.

Rossetti, L. (1986). *High-risk infants: Identification, assessment, and intervention.* Austin, TX: PRO-ED.

Schiefelbusch, R. L., & Lloyd, L. L. (Eds.). (1988). *Language perspectives: Acquisition, retardation, and intervention.* Austin, TX: PRO-ED.

Silverman, F. (1989). *Speech for the speechless.* Englewood Cliffs, NJ: Prentice-Hall.

Skinner, B. F. (1957). *Verbal behavior.* New York: Appleton-Century-Crofts.

Stoel-Gammon, C., & Dunn, C. (1985). *Normal and disordered phonology in children.* Austin, TX: PRO-ED.

Thompson, C. K. (1988). Articulation disorders in the child with neurogenic pathology. In N. J. Lass, L. V. McReynolds, J. L. Northern, & D. F. Yoder (Eds.), *Handbook of speech-language pathology & audiology* (pp. 548-591). Toronto, Canada: Decker

Tjossem, T. D. (Ed.). (1976). *Intervention strategies for high-risk infants and young children.* Baltimore: University Park Press.

Warren, S. F., & Rogers-Warren, A. K. (1985). *Teaching functional language.* Baltimore: University Park Press.

Weeks, M., & Gaylord-Ross, R. (1981). Task difficulty and aberrant behavior in severely handicapped students. *Journal of Applied Behavior Analysis, 14,* 449-463.

Wilson, D. K. (1987). *Voice disorders in children.* Baltimore: Williams & Wilkins.

Winokur, S. (1976). *A primer of verbal behavior.* Englewood Cliffs, NJ: Prentice-Hall.

Yorkston, K. M., Beukelman, D. R., & Bell, K. R. (1988). *Clinical management of dysarthric speakers.* Austin, TX: PRO-ED.

Appendix A

Glossary of Educational Abbreviations and Acronyms

The following is a list of acronyms and abbreviations commonly used in education. Additional or different acronyms and abbreviations may be used at specific school sites. The names of tests, associations, and universities have not been included in this list.

ADA: Average Daily Attendance
ADD: Attention Deficit Disorder
CA: Chronological Age
CH: Communicatively Handicapped
DD: Developmentally Disabled
DIS: Designated Instructional Service
ED: Emotionally Disturbed
            Department of Education
EDGAR: Education Department General Administrative Regulations
EEEA: Equity and Excellence in Education Act
EHA: Education for All Handicapped Children Act of 1975 (now known as IDEA as amended in 1990)
ESL: English as a Second Language
FAPE: Free Appropriate Public Education
FEP: Fluent-English Proficient

FERPA:	Family Education Rights and Privacy Act
FES:	Fluent-English Speaking
HBI:	Home-Based Instruction
HI:	Hearing Impaired
IDEA:	Individuals with Disabilities Education Act (1990 amendment of EHA changed name to IDEA)
IEP:	Individualized Education Program
IFSP:	Individualized Family Service Plan
IMC:	Instructional Materials (Media) Center
LD:	Learning Disability/Learning Disabled
LEA:	Local Education Agency
LEP:	Limited English Proficient
LES:	Limited English Speaking
LH:	Learning Handicapped
LRE:	Least Restrictive Environment
MA:	Mental Age
MR:	Mentally Retarded
NES:	Non-English Speaking
OCR:	Office For Civil Rights
OH:	Orthopedically Handicapped
OSEP:	Office of Special Education Programs, U.S. Department of Education (ED)
OSERS:	Office of Special Education and Rehabilitative Services, ED
OT:	Occupational Therapy
PL 94-142:	Public Law 94-142, The Education for all Handicapped Children Act of 1975
PL 99-457:	The 1986 amendments to the PL 94-142 which included the Early Intervention Program for Infants and Toddlers (Part H)
PLP:	Present Levels of Performance
RS:	Resource Specialist
SDC:	Special Day Class
SEA:	State Education Agency
SED:	Severely Emotionally Disturbed
SH:	Severely Handicapped
SST:	Student Study Team

Appendix B

Glossary of Medical Abbreviations and Symbols

Recording information in a patient's chart is a common form of communication among professionals in the medical setting. It provides a chronological log of patient services. Many abbreviations, acronyms, and symbols are used in recording data. Although there are universal symbols and abbreviations, some may be unique to a specific hospital. To avoid any misunderstanding, if you are unsure of an abbreviation, acronym, or symbol do not use it; instead, write out the entire word or phrase. Following is a list of some of the commonly used abbreviations, acronyms, and symbols. (Abbreviations for measurements, tests, and professional associations have not been included in this list.)

a.c.:   Before meals.
ACU: Ambulatory Care Unit or Acute Care Unit.
ACVD: Atherosclerotic Cardiovascular Disease.
AL: Allergy.
AMB: Ambulatory.
A/O: Alert and Oriented.
ASP: Aspirate.
b.i.d.:   Twice a day.
b.i.n.:   Twice a night.
c̄:   With.

CA: Cancer.
CHF: Congestive Heart Failure.
CHI: Closed Head Injury.
CNS: Central Nervous System.
CVA: Cerebral Vascular Accident.
DC (D/C):   Discontinue or Discharge.
Dx: Diagnosis.
h: Hour.
h.s.:   Hour of Sleep or Bedtime.
ICU: Intensive Care Unit.
Lt.:   Left.
NGT: Nasogastric Tube.
n.p.o.:   Nothing by mouth.
p.c.:   After meals.
p.o.:   By mouth.
p.r.n.:   As necessary.
pt.:   Patient.
q.:   Every.
q.d.:   Every day.
q.i.d.:   Four times a day.
Rt.:   Right.
Rx: Prescription or Therapy (Treatment).
s̄:   Without.
Stat.:   Immediately.
t.i.d.:   Three times a day.
t.i.n.:   Three times a night.
TPR: Temperature, Pulse, Respiration.
Tx: Therapy (Treatment).
♀   :Female.
♂   :Male.
↑   :Above or Increase.
↓   :Below or Decrease.
0   :Absent or No response.
ø   :No or None.
?   :Doubtful or Unknown-

Appendix C

Code of Ethics of the
American Speech-Language-Hearing Association
1991

Preamble

The preservation of the highest standards of integrity and ethical principles is vital to the successful discharge of the professional responsibilities of all speech-language pathologists and audiologists. This Code of Ethics has been promulgated by the Association in an effort to stress the fundamental rules considered essential to this basic purpose. Any action that is in violation of the spirit and purpose of this Code shall be considered unethical. Failure to specify any particular responsibility or practice in this Code of Ethics should not be construed as denial of the existence of other responsibilities or practices.

The fundamental rules of ethical conduct are described in three categories: Principles of Ethics, Ethical Proscriptions, Matters of Professional Propriety.

1. *Principles of Ethics.* Five Principles serve as a basis for the ethical evaluation of professional conduct and form the underlying moral basis for the Code of Ethics. Individuals[1] subscribing to this Code shall observe these principles as

---

[1] "Individuals" refers to all members of the American Speech-Language-Hearing Association and nonmembers who hold a Certificate of Clinical Competence from this Association.

affirmative obligations under all conditions of professional activity.

2. *Ethical Proscriptions.* Ethical Proscriptions are formal statements of prohibitions that are derived from the Principles of Ethics.

3. *Matters of Professional Propriety.* Matters of Professional Propriety represent guidelines of conduct designed to promote the public interest and thereby better inform the public and particularly the persons in need of speech-language pathology and audiology services as to the availability and the rules regarding the delivery of those services.

Principle of Ethics I

Individuals shall hold paramount the welfare of persons served professionally.

A. Individuals shall use every resource available, including referral to other specialists as needed, to provide the best service possible.

B. Individuals shall fully inform persons served of the nature and possible effects of these services.

C. Individuals shall fully inform subjects participating in research or teaching activities of the nature and possible effects of these activities.

D. Individuals' fees shall be commensurate with services rendered.

E.. Individuals shall provide appropriate access to records of persons served professionally.

F. Individuals shall take all reasonable precautions to avoid injuring persons in the delivery of professional services.

G. Individuals shall evaluate services rendered and products dispensed to determine effectiveness.

Ethical Proscriptions

1. Individuals must not exploit persons in the delivery of professional services, including accepting persons for treatment when benefit cannot reasonably be expected or continuing treatment unnecessarily.

2. Individuals must not guarantee the results of any therapeutic

procedures, directly or by implication. A reasonable statement of prognosis may be made, but caution must be exercised not to mislead persons served professionally to expect results that cannot be predicted from sound evidence.

3. Individuals must not use persons for teaching or research in a manner that constitutes invasion of privacy or fails to afford informed free choice to participate.

4. Individuals must not evaluate or treat speech, language or hearing disorders except in a professional relationship. They must not evaluate or treat solely by correspondence. This does not preclude follow-up correspondence with persons previously seen, nor providing them with general information of an educational nature.

5. Individuals must not reveal to unauthorized persons any professional or personal information obtained from the person served professionally, unless required by law or unless necessary to protect the welfare of the person or the community.

6. Individuals must not discriminate in the delivery of professional services on any basis that is unjustifiable or irrelevant to the need for and potential benefit from such services, such as race, sex, age, religion, national origin, sexual orientation, or handicapping condition.

7. Individuals must not charge for services not rendered.

Principle of Ethics II

Individuals shall maintain high standards of professional competence.

A. Individuals engaging in clinical practice or supervision thereof shall hold the appropriate Certificates(s) of Clinical Competence for the areas(s) in which they are providing or supervising professional services.

B. Individuals shall continue their professional development throughout their careers.

C. Individuals shall identify competent, dependable referrral sources for persons served professionally.

D. Individuals shall maintain adequate records of professional services rendered.

Ethical Proscriptions

1. Individuals must neither provide services nor supervision of services for which they have not been properly prepared, nor permit services to be provided by any of their staff who are not properly prepared.
2. Individuals must not provide clinical services by prescription of anyone who does not hold the Certificate of Clinical Competence.
3. Individuals must not delegate any service requiring the professional competence of a certified clinician to anyone unqualified.
4. Individuals must not offer clinical services by supportive personnel, students or clinical fellows for whom they do not provide appropriate supervision and assume full responsibility.
5. Individuals must not require anyone under their supervision to engage in any practice that is a violation of the Code of Ethics.

Principle of Ethics III

Individuals' statements to persons served professionally and to the public shall provide accurate information about the nature and management of communicative disorders, and about the profession and services rendered by its practitioners.

Ethical Proscriptions

1. Individuals must not misrepresent their training or competence.
2. Individuals' public statements providing information about professional services and products must not contain representations or claims that are false, deceptive or misleading.
3. Individuals must not use professional or commercial affiliations in any way that would mislead or limit services to persons served professionally.

Matters of Professional Propriety

1. Individuals should announce services in a manner consonant with highest professional standards in the community.

Principle of Ethics IV

Individuals shall honor their responsibilities to the public, their profession, and their relationships with colleagues and members of allied professions.

Ethical Proscriptions

1. Individuals must not participate in activities that constitute a conflict of professional interest.

Matters of Professional Propriety

1. Individuals should seek to provide and expand services to persons with speech, language, and hearing handicaps as well as to assist in establishing high professional standards for such programs.
2. Individuals should educate the public about speech, language, and hearing problems, and matters related to professional competence.
3. Individuals should strive to increase knowledge within the profession and share research with colleagues.
4. Individuals should establish harmonious relations with colleagues and members of other professions, and endeavor to inform members of related professions of services provided by speech-language pathologists and audiologists, as well as seek information from them.
5. Individuals should assign credit to those who have contributed to a publication in proportion to their contribution.
6. Individuals should not accept compensation for supervision or sponsorship from the clinical fellow being supervised or sponsored beyond reasonable reimbursement for direct expenses.
7. Individuals should present products they have developed to their colleagues in a manner consonant with highest professional standards.

Principle of Ethics V

Individuals shall uphold the dignity of the profession and freely accept the profession's self-imposed standards.

    A. Individuals shall inform the Ethical Practices Board when they have reason to believe that a member or certificate holder may have violated the Code of Ethics.

    B. Individuals shall cooperate fully with the Ethical Practice Board concerning matters of professional conduct related to this Code of Ethics.

Ethical Proscriptions

1. Individuals shall not engage in violations of the Principles of Ethics or in any attempt to circumvent any of them.
2. Individuals shall not engage in dishonesty, fraud, deceit, misrepresentation, or other forms of illegal conduct that adversely reflect on the profession or the individuals' fitness for membership in the profession.

Appendix D

Sample Clinical Interview

Interviewing Parents of a Stuttering Child

The following is a sample interview with parents of a 5-year-old stuttering child. Note the kinds of questions asked and the types of information sought by the clinician. Also, note how the clinician answered many questions the parents had about stuttering, its causes, and treatment.

Clinician: When did you first think that there may be something wrong with Brian's speech?

Mrs. Thomas: About a month ago, on a Sunday morning, I noticed that Brian was repeating a lot. I remember asking him what he wanted to eat for lunch that day. Brian started to say something like "I want a hot dog for lunch," but he had a lot of trouble saying it.

Clinician: What exactly did he do?

Mrs. Thomas: Well, he started like "I-I-I-I-I wa-wa-wa-want a hot d-d-d-d-dog, Mom." He was trying too hard to say it. I could see a lot of struggle to get it out.

Clinician: You had not heard that kind of problem in Brian's speech before?

Mr. Thomas: My wife has not heard it, but I have. About 2 months ago, when I was reading a story to him, he wanted to interrupt me to ask a question about the story. I don't remember what exactly he said at that time, but I remember him repeating a lot. Periodically I have heard him repeat a bit too much, but I thought it may be a passing thing. I remember him asking me once "What ta-ta-ta-time is it Dad?"

Clinician: Have you seen an increase in repetitions?

Mr. Thomas: I think so. During the last month or so, his speech problems have increased. He is repeating more and getting stuck more often. Now it takes him longer to get out of a block. And that, too, only after some struggle.

Clinician: What do you mean by a block?

Mrs. Thomas: His mouth and face look like he is trying hard to say something, but nothing comes out. His lips are quivering, mouth is sometimes open, at other times tightly shut. You can see the struggle to say something but he is not saying anything. This is what scares me the most.

Clinician: Did anything unusual happen around the time you first noticed his repetitions or more recently when you noticed an increase in them?

Mr. Thomas: No, not really. Things have been pretty routine at home.

Clinician: Has he been sick lately?

Mrs. Thomas: No, Brian has always been a healthy boy.

Clinician: What about your health when you were carrying Brian?

Mrs. Thomas: I was fine during pregnancy and the delivery was normal. The baby was healthy. We did not notice any problem until this stuttering came about.

Clinician: What about his speech and language development? Was there any reason to be concerned?

Mrs. Thomas: No. In fact, Brian began to speak earlier than my other son, Chad, who is 4 years older than him. We thought he was quite advanced in his speech. He usually talked a lot and learned new words fast.

Clinician: So everything has been normal until you began to notice his stuttering.

Mr. Thomas: We may have missed something, but that is our impression.

Clinician: I want to go back to Brian's stuttering. You said that he repeats a lot. Does he prolong a sound? Have you heard him say something like "I want sssssome ssssoup, please?" I prolonged the *s* sound in both the words. Does he prolong sounds like that?

Mrs. Thomas: Oh, yes. He does it all the time. This morning, while eating a new kind of cereal, he said "It is rad, Mom," but he prolonged the *a* sound. It was more like "raaaad."

Clinician: Does Brian repeat words and phrases? Does he say "I-I-I want it or let-let-let me do it or he-was he-was he-was coming" and things like that?

Mr. Thomas: Yes, we have heard him do that. Sometimes he repeats a word or a bunch of words many times before he moves on to the next word. Yesterday I heard him say to his brother "Why are you - why are you - why are you - why are you do- do - doing it?"

Clinician: Does he use what we call interjections like *uh* or *um* or *er*? As you know, most speakers have them, but I wonder how much Brian interjects.

Mrs. Thomas: I think he interjects a lot. In fact, Brian drives me up the wall with his *uhs* and *ums*. He starts a lot of sentences with ums. This morning he said "Um - um - um what am I - I - I g-g-g-going to have um - um - um - um for breakfast, Mom?" Sometimes he keeps going with ums.

Clinician: What about interjected words like *well, OK*, and phrases like *you know, I mean,* and *you see*?

Mrs. Thomas: He uses them some of the time. We hear more *ums* and *uhs* than what you just described.

Clinician: Does Brian show any facial grimaces when he stutters? Some people who stutter blink their eyes, wrinkle their noses and foreheads, purse their lips, wring their hands, swing their arms, and move their legs. Does Brian do any of these?

Mrs. Thomas: Yes, he does a few of those. I have seen him blink his eyes and wrinkle his nose and forehead. His hands and feet also move when he stutters. His mouth is distorted when he has a bad block. He also looks away from you when he stutters.

Clinician: Does Brian stutter all the time or only some of the time?

Mr. Thomas: His stuttering varies. One day we may hear just a few problems and the next day he may stutter on most of the words he speaks. He may be quite fluent in the morning but struggling to say his name in the afternoon. I find this puzzling. Is this true of other children who stutter, too?

Clinician: Yes, it is. A basic characteristic of stuttering is that it varies across time and speaking situations. Stuttering may be more when speaking on complex or unfamiliar topics. Dialogues in which one must take quick turns to talk and be silent also are difficult for stutterers. Stutterers are more fluent while talking aloud to themselves or when they are speaking in monologue. Stuttering also varies depending on the kinds of persons stutterers face. Stutterers may be very fluent talking to pets and babies. Many adult stutterers talk to their subordinates with increased fluency but when they confront their bosses, fluency may break down abruptly. Does Brian stutter more with some people and less with others?

Mr. Thomas: He is more fluent with his younger sister, Michelle, who is 3 years old. He has the most trouble with me, somewhat less with his mother. I would say his stuttering is about average when he talks to his older brother.

Mrs. Thomas: But his worst stuttering comes out when he talks to a stranger or in a new place. I took him to Chad's school the other day. One of the teachers there talked to Brian who blocked on every word he tried to say. The poor kid couldn't say his name. It was a heartbreaking scene for me. Also, his stuttering is worst when he talks to some of the kids in the neighborhood.

Clinician: Many stutterers avoid certain words. Older children and adults use substitutes for difficult words. Do you know of any words that Brian avoids saying?

Mrs. Thomas: I think I do. The other day Brian wouldn't say *John*, who is a friend of Chad. Brian kept saying "Your friend called" but wouldn't say who it was. When Chad asked about four times "Who was it?", Brian finally said "J-J-J-John" and stuttered very badly on it. Of late, I have not heard him say "Hi" to people because he can't get it out. Another puzzling thing about his problem is that he can sing songs and not have a trace of trouble. Is this also typical?

Clinician: Yes, it is! Most persons who stutter have no trouble singing.

Mr. Thomas: It's amazing! Though Brian has certain words on which he stutters frequently, he can say those very same words fluently. I suppose this is also characteristic of stuttering.

Clinician: That is also true. Stuttering on words is a matter of probability. Stuttering is more probable on some words than on other words. But even the words on which the stuttering probability is the highest may be, on occasion, spoken fluently. Therefore, it is not a question of not being able to say the words. As you know very well, Brian can say every word that he stutters on. He knows exactly what to say, he just cannot say it smoothly and easily.

Mrs. Thomas: That makes sense.

Clinician: I want to talk a little bit about the family history. Is there a history of speech disorders in the family? Are you aware of a speech problem on either side of the family?

Mr. Thomas: When I was a kid, I used to stutter. I do not believe that my father ever stuttered, but an uncle of mine did.

Clinician: Do you know when you began to stutter and how severe was it?

Mr. Thomas: I am not sure, but I think I began to stutter when I was about 4. I think it was pretty bad because I still remember having a lot of trouble in grade school. I remember the painful teasing and the frustration of getting blocked in front of the class and things like that.

Clinician: Did you receive treatment? Do you remember what it was?

Mr. Thomas: I did go to a speech therapist, but not very regularly. I can't remember much about what she did with me.

Clinician: When did your stuttering disappear, if it has. So far, you have not stuttered here.

Mr. Thomas: I do not stutter any more. I think my stuttering was at its peak during my years in intermediate school. High school was different. I began to experience more fluency, although I was not taking speech therapy at that time. The problem became less noticeable when I started college, and it disappeared in subsequent years. Is this common?

Clinician: To some degree. Persons who stutter may recover from it at any age, though recovery is more common in preschool children. Also, children who begin to stutter after age 7 also have a better chance of recovery. Children whose stuttering persists through the ages of 5 and 6 are likely to be chronic stutterers. During the early childhood years, girls who begin to stutter recover more often than boys of the same age. Roughly, some 30% of stutterers recover from it without much professional help. We call this **spontaneous recovery**. Mrs. Thomas, how about on your side of the family?

Mrs. Thomas: I do not believe there was a stutterer in my side of the family. I can't be sure, though. I did read in a newspaper article that stuttering runs in the family. Is this true?

Clinician: To a certain extent, stuttering tends to run in the family. The blood relatives of a stutterer have a greater chance of stuttering, compared to the blood relatives of nonstuttering persons. We call this the **familial incidence** of stuttering. But the higher familial incidence also is related to the **sex ratio**. You know that there are more male stutterers than female stutterers.

Mrs. Thomas: Yes, I have wondered about that. I have seen only one female stutterer in my life but many male stutterers. But how does it relate to the familial incidence?

Clinician: The familial incidence is related to the sex of one or more stutterers found in the family. If a male stutterer is found in a family, the familial incidence for that family may be higher compared to the incidence in the general population. However, if a female stutterer is found in a family, the familial incidence may be the highest. This means that though females are less likely to stutter, a stuttering female poses the maximum risk to the members of her family. In fact, the brothers and sons of a female stutterer run a very high risk of developing stuttering. Sisters and daughters of a stuttering male *or* female do not run that much of a risk. Of all the people, the sons of stuttering mothers run the greatest risk of developing stuttering.

Mr. Thomas: Does it mean that stuttering is hereditary?

Clinician: Some experts believe that stuttering is **genetically transmitted**, although the exact mechanism of transmission is not known. However, we must remember that all stutterers do not have stuttering relatives. Therefore, we cannot conclude that stuttering is inherited in all cases. Most experts believe that both heredity and environment play a role in the development of stuttering.

Mrs. Thomas: If it is inherited, is it more difficult to treat?

Clinician: No, there are no data that suggest that. Research has shown that almost all stutterers improve under treatment and many to a significant extent. Early treatment of stuttering is especially effective and I am glad that you brought Brian in this early.

Mr. Thomas: Well that is good news for Brian and for us!

Appendix E

Examples of Dysfluency Types

Dysfluency types	Examples
REPETITIONS:	
Part-word repetitions	"What *ta-ta-ta*-time is it?"
Whole-word repetitions	"*What-what-what* are you doing?"
Phrase repetitions	"*I want to-I want to-I want to* do it"
PROLONGATIONS:	
Sound/syllable prolongations	"*Lllllet* me do it."
Silent prolongations	A struggling attempt to say a word when there is no sound.
INTERJECTIONS:	
Sound/syllable interjections	"*um...um* I had a problem this morning."
Whole-word interjections	"I had a *well* problem this morning."
Phrase interjections	"I had a *you know* problem this morning."
SILENT PAUSES	
A silent duration within speech considered abnormal	"I was going to the (pause) store."

BROKEN WORDS
A silent pause within words: "It was won(pause)derful."

INCOMPLETE PHRASES
Grammatically incomplete   *"I don't know how to...* Let us
utterances   go, guys."

REVISIONS
Changed words, ideas   "I thought I will write a letter, card."

How to Calculate Percentage Dysfluency Rates

Measure the frequency of all types of dysfluencies exhibited in a sample. Count the number of words spoken in the sample. Calculate the percentage dysfluency rate as shown in the following example.

Types of Dysfluency	Frequency
Part-word repetitions	19
Whole word repetitions	12
Phrase repetitions	22
Silent prolongations	34
Sound prolongations	26
Sound/syllable interjections	21
Word interjections	13
Phrase interjections	16
Broken words	10
Silent pauses	17
Incomplete phrases	9
Revisions	2
Total of all types	201
Number of words spoken	978
Percent dysfluency rate	**20.5**

$$\left(\frac{201}{978} \times 100 = 20.5\%\right)$$

Appendix F

Obtaining and Analyzing
Conversational Speech Samples

The conversational speech sample provides data essential to the evaluation of your clients' articulation, fluency, voice, and language. The following information provides guidelines for obtaining and analyzing conversational speech samples of children and adults.

Obtaining Speech Samples

1. Obtain a representative sample of your clients' speech. Obtain a minimum of 100 utterances. An extended sample of 300 to 500 utterances is preferred. It is necessary to sample conversation in a variety of environments with different individuals. Ask clients to bring in a taped sample of their speech at home, work, or school. Tell them that while taping, they should be doing most of the talking. With very young children, or children with severely limited speech and language, you may need to sample speech over several sessions. If you are unable to adequately sample a child's speech, ask the parent to maintain a record of the child's speech for one week. Schedule another session in which you evoke speech from the child. If the child is reluctant to talk with you, obtain a sample of the child's speech while he or she talks with the parent.

Explain to parents that you want them to talk with the child as they normally would while you are out of the room. Record the conversation.

2. Video tape-record the sample if possible. You will be able to review nonverbal behaviors later. In addition to speech, you will be able to note eye contact, gestures, attention to tasks, and so on. You also may observe if your change in posture or position affects the client's communicative behaviors.

3. Audio tape-record the sample if video recording is not available or practical. Attach a small clip-on microphone to your client's collar if he or she will be sitting in the same place throughout the sample. (This usually results in better quality recording of the client's voice.) Have a paper and pen available to note any relevant nonverbal behaviors.

4. Check your recording equipment before beginning your session. Make sure your equipment is operating correctly. Check batteries, electrical plugs and outlets, and tapes. Turn equipment on before beginning your sample.

5. Have a variety of materials available. Different children, adolescents, and adults have different interests. Have different types and sizes of toys available for children (e.g., large and small blocks, trucks, and dolls). Have different types of pictures available (e.g., pictures of sports activities, children playing, and people crying, laughing, and yelling).

6. Engage adults and adolescents in conversation. You usually do not need to use stimulus materials with them. Often the interview will allow you to obtain one conversational sample. Later you can ask them to talk on the phone, talk with the secretary, or speak with another clinician. You occasionally may need to use such materials as pictures with adolescents.

7. Try and engage children in conversation before bringing out books and toys. Many children will talk to the clinician if they are given the chance. Do not bring out toys and books until after you first have tried to engage the child in a conversation. Talk with a child about least and favorite school activities, cartoons, movies, vacations, friends, pets, teachers, birthdays and other special occasions, and so forth. Discuss likes and dislikes about siblings, and events that make them very happy, mad, or sad. (If a child's speech is unintelligible, you may have to use props to try and understand his or her speech.)

8. Avoid using books. Unless you plan to have a client retell the story, do not use books. Children want to look at the pictures

or read the books, rather than describe what is happening in the pictures.

9. Keep questions to a minimum. Use open-ended statements such as: *Tell me about your classes, Tell me about your favorite TV show.* Avoid asking closed-end questions such as: *Are you taking a math class? Is your birthday coming?*

10. Tell something about yourself. For example, if you know a child has a sister, talk about your sister first: *My sister really made me upset yesterday. She wouldn't let me watch the TV show that I wanted to watch.* Talk about a recent movie you know the child has seen: *I went to see Batman last night, but, you know what? I fell asleep and don't know how it ended!"*

11. Allow children to direct the conversation. You may present a subject or activity and the child may have a completely different idea of what he or she wants to discuss. Follow the child's lead in beginning communications. You can always direct the conversation later to sample additional language structures.

12. Give opportunities for the client to exhibit different language structures. Direct the conversation to allow the client to talk about past, present, and future occurrences. Sample the use of pronouns, declaratives, interrogatives, negation, and so on.

13. Allow pauses in the conversation. Don't worry if there are periods of silence in your client interaction. Allow your clients plenty of time to respond to questions. Give them time to continue the conversation.

14. Relax and have fun with children. Children like such absurdities as boxes that "talk," balls that bounce to the moon, and puppets that have squeaky voices.

Analyzing Speech Samples

1. Transcribe the conversational speech sample as soon as possible. Allow sufficient time to record all necessary information.

2. Transcribe the sample using standard English orthography. It is unnecessary to transcribe an entire sample phonetically. Transcribe unintelligible utterances and misarticulated words phonetically.

3. Record context in which speech is produced. Include in your transcription events preceding each of the client's utterances. For example, if you showed a picture, asked a question, discussed an event, or performed an action, include this as part of your transcription: *Clinician: bounced the ball. Client: "Pretty ball."*

4. Include in your analysis, mean length of utterance, and syntactic, morphologic, semantic, and pragmatic use. As much as possible, give percentage of occurrences. Describe how many production opportunities (obligatory contexts) were present for a particular feature and in how many of those opportunities the feature was used correctly. For instance, a child may have had 20 opportunities to produce the regular plural morpheme but may have produced it correctly in only 10 of them. This means the child's correct production of the regular plural morpheme is 50%. Try to give such quantitative data for language structures of interest.

5. Analyze voice characteristics including pitch, rate, and intensity. These may be statements of clinical judgments unless a disorder is noted.

6. Analyze fluency. Describe all dysfluency forms and calculate total percentage of dysfluencies.

7. Compute speech intelligibility. Overall speech intelligibility may be computed using the total conversational speech sample, rather than the sample for language analysis. Some language analysis programs exclude unintelligible utterances from the analysis. Note if any articulation errors produced at the conversation level are different from, or in addition to, those noted in single-word productions.

8. Save your conversational speech analysis to compare with later samples.

Appendix G

Sample Probe Recording Sheet

The following shows the probe procedure in which the trained (T) and untrained (U) responses (preposition *on* in phrases) are alternated to find out the percentage correct probe response rate.

Client: Javier Nunez   Clinician: Nittur Chand
Age: 8   Date: 5-5-92
Disorder: Language   Session No. 7
Target Behavior: Preposition Reinforcement: Verbal; for
  on in phrases   the trained responses only

Target Behaviors	Scoring
1. Juice on table **(T)**	+
2. Pillow on sofa (U)	+
3. Dog on floor **(T)**	+
4. Man on horse (U)	−
5. Woman on bike **(T)**	+
6. Boy on skateboard (U)	+
7. Girl on roof **(T)**	−
8. Cookie on counter (U)	+

Target Behaviors	Scoring
9. Pot on stove **(T)**	+
10. Pen on desk (U)	–
11. Clock on wall **(T)**	+
12. Ball on chair (U)	+
13. Teddy on bed **(T)**	+
14. Book on shelf (U)	+
15. Hat on head **(T)**	+
16. Baby on shoulders (U)	+
17. Spot on shirt **(T)**	+
18. Wrinkle on face (U)	–
19. Cat on tree **(T)**	+
20. Bird on tree (U)	+

Note: (+) = Correct   (–) = Incorrect
Percentage Correct Probe Response Rate: 70

In this example, 10 trained exemplars were intermixed with 10 untrained exemplars. Responses given to trained exemplars were reinforced while those given to untrained exemplars were not. In calculating the percentage correct probe response rate, responses given to only the untrained exemplars are considered. The client's responses to 7 of the 10 untrained exemplars were correct, yielding a 70% correct probe response rate for the production of preposition *on* in phrases.

Appendix H

Treatment Plans

Treatment plans provide a comprehensive program of treatment from the beginning of treatment to dismissal. Treatment plans are developed before beginning treatment and can be modified, if necessary, as treatment progresses. Following is a sample of a Treatment Plan.

University Speech and Hearing Clinic
Treatment Plan

Name: Oliver Driver
Address: 312 N. South #111
City: Martinsville, 64812
Telephone: 782-9832
School: Preschool

Date of Birth: February 1, 1986
File no.: 900111-3
Diagnosis: Articulation
Semesters in Therapy: 1
Date of Report: June 19, 1990

Background Information
Oliver Driver, a 4-year-old-male, began his first semester of speech treatment at the University Speech and Hearing Clinic on February 1, 1990. Oliver's speech and language were evaluated on January 15, 1990. The evaluation revealed an articulation disorder characterized by substitutions, omissions, and reduced intelligibility. See his folder for a diagnostic report. Treatment was recommended to train correct production of misarticulated phonemes to increase speech intelligibility.

Target Behavior

Based on inconsistent production during assessment, the production of the following phonemes was selected for the initial treatment: /p/, /m/, /s/, /k/, and /g/. Production of each phoneme was baserated with 20 stimulus words administered on modeled and evoked discrete trials. Oliver's correct production of the target phonemes on modeled and evoked baserate trials were as follows:

/p/: 15%
/m/: 10%
/s/: 22%
/k/: 18%
/g/: 14%

Treatment was begun after obtaining the baserates. The following general treatment procedures will be used during the semester. The procedures will be modified as suggested by Oliver's performance data. These changes will be described in the final summary report.

Treatment Procedure

Training for each target phoneme will begin at the word level. When Oliver's probe response rate at the word level meets a 90% correct criterion, training will be initiated on two-word phrases. A similar probe criterion will be used to shift training to sentences and then to conversational speech.

Intermixed probes on which trained and untrained words, phrases, or sentences are alternated will be administered every time Oliver meets a tentative training criterion of 90% correct response rate on a block of 20 evoked training trials. Oliver will be trained to meet this criterion at each level of response topography (words, phrases, sentences).

Initially, the clinician will provide stimulus pictures, but Oliver will be required to find at least five pictures in magazines or draw two pictures representing the target sound and bring them to the clinic sessions. After he correctly produces the target sound on five consecutive trials, he will paste the pictures in a book to be used for both clinic and home practice.

Training will begin at each level with discrete trials and modeling. The clinician will show Oliver a picture, ask a question ("What is this?") and model the response (word or phrase). Oliver will then be required to imitate the clinician's production. When Oliver correctly imitates the target sound on five consecutive trials, modeling will be discontinued. The clinician will show Oliver a picture and ask "What is this?" to evoke a response.

At the modeled and evoked word levels, verbal reinforcement will be administered on an FR1 schedule for correct productions. At the phrase and sentence levels, a FR4 will be used. At the conversational level verbal reinforcement will be delivered on an approximate VR5 schedule. All incorrect productions at each level will immediately be interrupted by saying "stop."

Modeling will be reintroduced if Oliver gives two to four incorrect responses on the evoked trials. Shaping with manual guidance will be used as necessary.

All productions will be charted by the clinician. Oliver also will chart productions with an X under the "happy face" or X under the "sad face." At the end of each session, Oliver will assist the clinician in recording his progress on a graph.

It is expected that different target sounds will reach the training criterion at different times. Therefore, the clinician expects to train several sounds at different response topographies in each session. Some sounds may be trained at the word level while others may be trained at the phrase or even sentence level. When the initially selected target sounds meet the criterion of 90% correct probe rate in conversational speech in the clinic, new target sounds will be baserated and trained.

Maintenance Program
After Oliver produces the target sound with 90% accuracy at the evoked word level, his mother will be asked to participate in treatment. Initially, she will observe the treatment procedure, and then she will present stimulus items and chart correct and incorrect productions. She will be trained to immediately reinforce the correct productions and stop Oliver at the earliest sign of an inaccurate production.

After Oliver's mother identifies correct and incorrect responses with at least 90% accuracy in the clinic session, she will be trained to work with him at home. The mother will begin with such structured activities as reciting from a list or "reading" from the book he is developing in treatment. Assignments will progress to monitoring and recording speech during dinner and phone conversations with Oliver's grandmother. She will be trained to prompt and then praise the correct productions in conversational speech. Oliver, the clinician, and Oliver's mother will review tape-recorded home assignments. The mother will be given feedback on the procedures implemented at home

When Oliver produces the target sound with 90% accuracy in conversation in the sessions, he will be taken out of the clinic to practice correct productions in nonclinical situations. The clinician will take Oliver for a walk on campus and talk with him. Subsequently, he may be taken to the campus bookstore, library, cafeteria, and other places. Eventually, his speech may be monitored informally in shopping centers and restaurants.

When Oliver's speech is 98% intelligible and he produces most of his speech sounds at least 90% correct, he may be dismissed from treatment. A follow-up visit will be scheduled for 6 months after dismissal. Based on the initial follow-up results, booster treatment, treatment for persistent errors, or additional follow-ups will be planned.

Marla Model, Student Clinician

Barbara Sierra, M.S., CCC/SLP
Clinical Supervisor

Appendix I

Lesson Plan

Lesson plans describe what the clinician intends to do in a treatment session. Lesson plans may be brief or detailed depending on the site and your supervisor. In all cases, lesson plans should give enough information so your supervisor can understand and evaluate them.

UNIVERSITY SPEECH AND HEARING CLINIC
LESSON PLAN

Client: Erik Sounds   Age: 6-3
Clinician: Julie Matters   Supervisor: Wendy Marks
Date: 9/10/91

Objective: *Production of initial /l/ with 90% accuracy at word level in nonimitated training trials.*

Procedures: *I will present pictures of words representing /l/ in the initial position. In the beginning, I will model the correct productions. When Erik imitates at 90% accuracy in at least 10 trials, I will skip modeling and ask him to name the pictures. I will reinforce each*

279

correct production with verbal praise. I will stop Erik every time he begins to produce an incorrect response by saying "no" or "stop." Toward the end of the session, Erik will begin to plot his progress on a chart.

Results:

Objective: *Correct production of /f/ in conversational speech with 95% accuracy in all word positions.*

Procedures: *I will ask Erik to talk about the baseball game he is going to next week. If he has difficulty thinking of things to say, I will prompt him with pictures of baseball games. I will reinforce his correct production on a FR5 schedule. I will react to his incorrect production as described before. I will ask him to self-correct all incorrect /f/ productions in conversational speech.*

Results:

Appendix J

Diagnostic Report

NAME: Susan Mason

BIRTHDATE: February 8, 1970
AGE: 28
ADDRESS: 44 W. Wilson
CITY: Lothar
TELEPHONE: 448-3312
REFERRED BY: Dr. Marie Meyr

DATE OF EVALUATION:
February 9, 1991
DIAGNOSIS: Voice Disorder
EXAMINER: Dawn Goode
SUPERVISOR: Faye Kremtolf
INFORMANT: Self
OCCUPATION: Student
FILE NO: 91032-51

Statement of Problem

Susan Mason, a 21-year-old female, was seen for a speech and language evaluation at the University Speech and Hearing Clinic. Susan was referred to the university clinic by Dr. Marie Meyr, an otolaryngologist. Susan reported difficulty speaking for long periods of time. Susan said that Dr. Meyr had diagnosed vocal nodules.

Background Information

Susan's medical history was unremarkable with the exception of the recent diagnosis of vocal nodules. In a report dated December 2, 1990, Dr. Meyr stated the presence of "bilateral vocal nodules in the classical osition." Dr. Meyr recommended surgical intervention for removal of the nodules; however, Susan chose not to follow the recommendations. Subsequently, Dr. Meyr recommended voice evaluation and treatment at the University Speech and Hearing Clinic

Susan reported that she majored in economics and was active on a livestock judging team. She stated that judging took place from October to April, during which time she practiced 3 to 4 hours daily. On judging days, Susan was required to use her voice almost continually for 7 hours. She reported that she must use a louder than normal intensity level during judging. According to Susan, her voice did not interfere with her ability to communicate with others; however, she was concerned about the sound of her voice and how quickly her voice fatigued. She reported that in Sept. 1990, while yelling, she experienced a sharp pain in the laryngeal area. This experience had frightened her and she sought medical help.

Susan further reported that her voice sounds much better in the mornings and on days when she does not speak much. But often, by evening her voice is hoarse and tired.

Observations and Assessment Results

Oral peripheral: An oral peripheral examination revealed relatively symmetrical facial features and adequate labial and lingual movement. Palatal structures were within normal limits. Adequate velopharyngeal functions were noted. The soft palate elevated symmetrically upon phonation of /a/. Velopharyngeal closure was acoustically judged to be within normal limits. Normal muscular function was demonstrated during rapid articulatory movement.

Hearing: A pure tone audiometric screening was performed at 15 dB HTL for the frequencies 500, 1000, 2000, and 4000 Hz. Bilateral responses were obtained for all frequencies.

Articulation: Articulation was evaluated during Susan's spontaneous speech and reading of the "Rainbow Passage." Speech was 100% intelligible. No articulation errors were noted.

Language: An analysis of a 100-utterance language sample did not reveal any deviations. The mean length of utterance was 7.5 words and 8.0 morphemes. All language structures were correctly used.

Fluency: The conversational speech sample was used to assess fluency and dysfluencies. Susan's dysfluency rate was 3% and consisted mainly of syllable and word interjections. Her rate and types of dysfluencies were not of clinical significance.

Voice: A conversational speech sample of 250 words was obtained to evaluate overall vocal quality. Vocal quality was characterized by inappropriately loud intensity, hoarseness, low pitch, and pitch breaks. Frequent hard glottal attacks and throat clearing were observed throughout the assessment session.

Susan spoke in a loud voice during the evaluation. Sound level meter measurements revealed speech consistently exceeding 60 dB. When asked to lower her intensity, Susan did so for four or five words, then gradually increased her intensity. Susan said that she used a loud voice in other environments. She stated that her roommate had told her not to bother to use the telephone because her voice was so loud she didn't need one.

Chest and clavicular breathing were observed throughout the assessment. Maximum duration of phonation and breath support were measured by having Susan prolong the phoneme /a/. Susan exhibited the ability to sustain /a/ for 5, 7, and 6 seconds over three separate trials, well below the optimal level of 16 seconds. Three separate trials were used to measure Susan's ability to sustain the cognates /s/ and /z/. The average ratio for these trials was 0.70 which was below the expected level of 1.0 for normal speakers. A reading sample also revealed inefficient breath support. In reading, 80% of Susan's phrases deteriorated into glottal fry or hoarseness by the second word of the phrase.

Habitual pitch was measured using the Visi-Pitch. Habitual pitch during conversational speech was 196 Hz, with a pitch range of 57.8 Hz to 988 Hz. The higher frequencies were noted during pitch breaks. Variable pitch and frequent pitch breaks were noted frequently during spontaneous speech. Optimal pitch was determined to be 262 Hz. Susan could increase her pitch using feedback from the Visi-Pitch. When pitch was raised, hoarseness was eliminated until pitch again decreased.

Rate, resonance, and inflection were evaluated during conversation. These vocal parameters were considered normal.

Summary of Findings

Susan Mason's otolaryngologist has diagnosed bilateral vocal nodules. The current voice assessment suggests a history of vocal abuse, and that her voice is inappropriately loud and characterized by hoarseness, low pitch, and frequent pitch breaks. Susan exhibited inefficient breath support during phonation and employed several vocally abusive speech behaviors.

Recommendations

It is recommended that Susan Mason receive speech-language pathology services for treatment of her voice disorder, a minimum of two sessions per week. Treatment should focus on eliminating vocally abusive behaviors, increasing breath support, and increasing pitch. It is also recommended that Susan return to her otolaryngologist for a follow-up visit after 3 months of voice treatment at this clinic.

_____

Dawn Goode, Student Clinician

_____

Faye Kremtolf, M.A., CCC/SLP
Clinical Supervisor

Appendix K

Discrete Trial Treatment Procedure and Recording Form

In the discrete trial treatment procedure, you may use two to six training stimuli at any one time. The following example shows how to train the present progressive *ing* using modeling and six exemplars (training stimuli). Skip modeling according to the criteria described in the text.

1. Place the stimulus picture in front of the client. For example, place the picture of a *boy running* in front of the client.
2. Ask a question designed to evoke the correct response. Ask "What is the boy doing?"
3. Immediately model the correct response. Say, *"the boy is running."*
4. Wait a few seconds for the client to respond.
5. If the response is correct, immediately reinforce the client. If the response is incorrect (the present progressive omitted), say "No" and use other response reduction procedures (token loss, time-out).
6. Record the response on your recording sheet.
7. Pull the stimulus picture away from the client to mark the end of the trial.
8. Start the next trial by placing the picture in front of the client again.

Discrete Trial Treatment Recording Sheet

In the following example, the clinician trained a person with aphasia in naming five photographs or pictures and recorded the responses on the recording sheet. On discrete trials, modeling was introduced and withdrawn as shown.

Client: Wendy Nullnem
Age: 65
Disorder: Aphasia
Target Behavior: Naming

Clinician: Arnold Chatters
Date: 3-3-92
Session No. 5
Reinforcement: Continuous/Verbal

Target Responses   Blocks of 10 Training Trials

	1	2	3	4	5	6	7	8	9	10	% Correct
1. "Tom"	m+	−	+	−	−	+	−	+	+	+	
(Husband)	+	+	e−	−	m+	+	e+	+	+	+	m 71%/e 83%
2. "Jenny"	m+	+	−	+	−	+	+	+	−+	+	
(Daughter)	e−	−	m+	+	e+	+	+	−	+	+	m 83%/e 62%
3. "Cup"	m−	+	−	+	−	+	+	+	−	+	
	+	+	+	+	e+	−	+	+	−	+	m 71% /e 66%
4. "Water"	m+	+	−	+	+	−	+	+	+	+	
	+	e−	−	m+	+	+	+	e+	+	+	m 86%/e 60%
5. "Phone"	m−	+	+	+	+	+	e−	−	m+	+	
	e−	+	−	+	+	−	+	−+	−+	+	m 85% /e 58%

Note: (+) = Correct response (−) = Incorrect or no response
       m = Modeled trial e = Evoked trial, no modeling
       Total Number of trials: _____
       Total % Correct Responses: _____

Appendix L

Daily Progress Notes

Progress notes are recorded after each treatment session to document client progress. Following is a sample of progress notes using "SOAP notes" (subjective, objective, assessment, plan).

CITY HOSPITAL SPEECH-LANGUAGE PATHOLOGY AND AUDIOLOGY DEPARTMENT

Name of patient:
Date of birth:
Clinician(s)

Date	Progress Notes	Initials

9/23/91 John appeared alert today. He greeted the clinician with a smile. The client responded to 20 yes/no questions with 70% accuracy. He produced simple CV words @ the imitation level with 80% accuracy. John demonstrated progress in both Treatment tasks today. Response to yes/no questions ↑ 60% to 70% (in 20 trials). Imitative productions ↑ from 75% to 80% for CV words. Continue current activities · APG SP /////

Date	Progress Notes	Initials

9/24/91 John greeted the clinician c̄ a smile, but appeared tired – his eyes closed occasionally during the 30 minute session. Client responded to yes/no questions c̄ 70%. Imitative tasks for CV words was 60%. John demonstrated ↓ in both tasks today. As noted, he seemed tired. This was discussed c̄ nurse who reported that John had not slept well. Rec. continue current activities, but re-eval if John's behavior/health changes.

SPG SP /////

Appendix M

Sample Progress Report

May 26, 1991
Richard Smith, M.D.
3030 E. Fairview Ave., #24
Oceanview, CA 93711

SPEECH-LANGUAGE PROGRESS REPORT
PATIENT: John North
DOB: 02/10/88
PERIOD COVERED: 11/25/90 - 05/25/91
NUMBER OF SESSIONS ATTENDED: 42
LENGTH OF SESSIONS: 30 MINUTES EACH

Background Information
John North, a 3-year, 3-month-old boy was seen for a speech and language evaluation on August 16, 1990. The evaluation revealed significantly delayed speech and language with verbal apraxia. At that time, John was basically nonverbal with the exception of a few single syllable word approximations. He had less than 15 functional words. As a result of the evaluation, John was enrolled in speech-language treatment. He received treatment approximately twice a week from November 25, 1991 to May 25, 1991.

Summary of Treatment

Goal 1: Production of the following sounds with at least 90% accuracy in conversational speech in the clinic and home setting: /p, b, m, n, t, d, k, g/, and /s/.

Treatment: Treatment began at the phoneme level for each sound and progressed to the word, phrase, and conversation level after a criteria of 95% accuracy was met at each level. Tactile, auditory, and visual stimulation initially were used to train sound production. Verbal praise and token gain and loss were used during treatment.

Progress: This goal has been met.

Goal 2: Production of the following language features in continuous speech during structured treatment activities with 90% accuracy: present progressive, regular plural morphemes, posessives, regular past tense inflections, and prepositions.

Treatment: John was presented with stimulus pictures representing each word in the phrase. The clinician modeled each phrase and John was required to touch each card as he imitated the clinician (e.g., boy is jumping). John was praised for his correct productions. Incorrect productions were interrupted and the clinician modeled the correct production.

Progress: John met the goal for the following structures: present progressive, plurals, posessives, and the prepositions "in," "on," and "under." John continues to work on the regular past tense.

Impressions and Recommendations
John has made excellent progress in his speech and language treatment sessions. His willingness to try and interact with others and the reinforcement of successful communication have had a positive effect on his behavior and social development. Excellent parental support and participation from his mother has encouraged carry-over into other environments. John is now able to communicate using a larger vocabulary of single words and simple sentences of two to three words. It is recommended that John continue to receive speech-language services two times per week. Treatment will emphasize the following:

1. Continued training on the regular past tense.
2. Production of the following sounds: /f, w, ng, y, sh/, and /l/.

3. Increased mean length of utterance.
4. Parent training to work with John at home.

I hope this information is helpful. Please contact me if you have questions.

Susan Frances, M.A., CCC-SLP

Appendix N

Final Summary

The final summary is written at the end of a treatment period (such as at the end of the semester). It provides information on the client's treatment, progress, and recommendations for continuing treatment. Following is a sample of a Final Summary.

University Speech and Hearing Clinic
FINAL SUMMARY

Client: John Gill
Address: 444 E. Southdrive
City: Grayson
Telephone: 610-3456
Occupation: Student
Period Covered: February 1,
  1991 - May 1, 1991

Birthdate: January 1, 1966
Clinic File No.: 910077
Diagnosis: Fluency
Semester in Clinic: 1
Date of Report: May 1, 1991

Clinic Schedule
Sessions per week: 2
Number of clinic visits: 22

Length of sessions: 1 hour
Total clinic hours: 22 hours

Status at the Beginning of Treatment
John Gill, a 25-year-old male, began his first semester of treatment at the

University Speech and Hearing Clinic. John reported that he stuttered. He said it interfered with his part-time job as a store clerk and that people occasionally made fun of his speech. He reported that he had received speech therapy when he was 9 and 10 years old, but that he always continued to stutter.

Two conversational speech samples were analyzed before beginning treatment. Language, voice, and articulation were subjectively evaluated and judged to be normal. The first sample, obtained in the clinic, contained 1,400 words. The percentage dysfluency rate for this sample was 18%. The second sample was recorded by John when he talked with his wife at home. This sample revealed a dysfluency rate of 16%. Both samples contained part-word repetitions, whole-word repetitions, interjections of words and phrases, pauses, and prolongations. A complete diagnostic report dated February 1, 1991 is placed in the folder.

Summary of Treatment

Treatment involved training fluent speech through the use of a management of airflow, easy vocal onset, and reduced rate of speech through vowel prolongation. A detailed treatment program written for John may be found in the folder.

Initially, each of the fluency skills were trained separately. John was asked to inhale a larger than the usual amount of air, immediately exhale a small amount of air through his mouth, and begin saying the word in a soft and easy manner. He was asked to prolong the vowels and speak at a reduced rate. This process usually resulted in stutter-free speech.

Stutter-free speech was trained starting with words and phrases. In gradual steps, treatment progressed to controlled sentences and conversational speech. In all treatment sessions, the criterion of fluency required of John was 98% or better. Both dysfluencies and errors in fluency skills (e.g., failure to inhale or exhale, abrupt phonatory onset, rapid rate) were measured in all sessions. When John maintained at least 98% fluent speech at any level of training for either a block of 50 utterances (phrases, sentences) or for a duration of 10 minutes or more, the training was moved to the next level of response topography. If John's dysfluency rate increased when moved to a higher level of training, he was returned to the lower level.

At the earliest sign of an incorrect response or a dysfluency, John was asked to "Stop." In the initial stages, he was told what went wrong. For example, the clinician said: "You forgot to breathe in"; "You did not breathe out;" "You were about to stutter"; and so forth. Later on, he was asked simply to "Stop." Correct productions of target behaviors resulting in stutter-free speech were verbally reinforced at the end of the response chain. Initially, a continuous schedule was used; gradually, the amount of reinforcement was reduced to an approximate VR5 schedule at the conversational level.

John was trained to chart the correct use of target behaviors and all dysfluencies. After John demonstrated accurate monitoring of responses and 98% fluency at each level, home assignments were given for that level. John's wife observed four sessions in which she was trained to monitor his fluent speech by stopping and reinforcing him as the clinician did. John and his wife were recommended to practice the skills of fluency for at least 20 minutes each day. John's wife was asked also to monitor his speech in most speaking situations.

To promote maintenance, the clinician accompanied John to the campus book store and cafeteria where he talked to other persons. The clinician monitored John's speech by giving subtle hints to prompt the target responses and provided verbal reinforcement whenever practical. Various probes were taken to document changes in his dysfluency rate.

Results

By the end of the semester, John's fluency rate in conversational speech with the clinician at the clinic was 98%. However, a 10-minute conversational speech sample recorded at his home with his wife showed a fluency rate of 94%. A probe of his speech with his boss at work showed a fluency rate of 92%.

Recommendations

It is recommended that John continue treatment for his stuttering. The treatment next semester should emphasize maintenance of fluency at home, office, and other settings.

Dana Monroe, Student Clinician

Greg Hallstoni, M.S., CCC/SLP
Clinical Supervisor

Appendix O

Sample Referral Letters

Speech-language pathologists write many kinds of referral letters to other professionals. The following three kinds are common.

REFERRAL LETTER 1
The following sample illustrates the kind of letter a speech-language pathologist might write to another professional to acknowledge the referral of a client for speech-language services.

August 10, 1991

John Ellis, M.D.
228 N. Way, Suite 101
Bloomington, CO 78123

Dear Dr. Ellis:

Thank you for referring Oliver Colby to our Clinic. He was seen for a speech and language evaluation on August 5, 1991. Oliver was accompanied to the evaluation by his mother who expressed concern over her son's lack of speech intelligibility.

Results of the assessment revealed a severe articulation disorder, with multiple sound substitutions and omissions. Receptive language was age appropriate; however, expressive language was delayed. Oliver was cooperative during the evaluation and easily stimulable for the sounds he misarticulated and omitted.

I recommended that Oliver begin treatment for his speech and language disorder. He will be seen two times per week for one hour each visit.

Enclosed is a copy of Oliver's speech and language evaluation report. If you have any questions, please contact me at 581-2285.

Sincerely,

Dorothy Jacobson, M.A., CCC/SLP
Speech-LanguagePathologist

REFERRAL LETTER 2
The following sample illustrates the kind of letter one speech-language pathologist might write to another to make a referral.

May 10, 1991
Donna Jones, M.S.
Speech-Language Pathologist
Melvin Communication Clinic
Melvin, Alaska

Dear Ms. Jones:

Robert Fine, a 67-year-old man, who suffered a stroke nearly four months ago was diagnosed with apraxia and aphasia, characterized by moderate auditory comprehension and severe verbal expression deficits. At the time of assessment, his conversational speech consisted primarily of several automatic phrases.

Robert has received treatment at our clinic for the past three months. He has demonstrated significant progress. He is able to express himself in 6- to 7-word utterances. He accurately uses many language structures including nouns, various verb tenses, modifiers, plurals, possessives, and some prepositional phrases.

Though Robert has made good progress, he needs continued treatment to stabilize his conversational speech skills in extraclinical situations. Because he is moving to your town, I am referring him to your clinic. Robert is highly motivated to continue treatment. He would be an excellent candidate for your treatment program. I hope you will consider accepting Robert as a client. If you have questions, please contact me at 292-8888.

Sincerely,

Georgia Surr, M.S., CCC/SLP

REFERRAL LETTER 3
The following sample illustrates the kind of letter a speech-language pathologist might write to a physician (or another professional) to refer a client.

July 15, 1991
Jean Griffin, M.D.
333 W. Hills, Suite 101
Beverly, NM 20111

Dear Dr. Griffin,

I saw Jerry Blank in my office for a voice evaluation on July 1, 1991. He requested an evaluation because he felt that his voice was "too deep." During the evaluation he reported chronic hoarseness and occasional pain in the laryngeal area.

During the voice evaluation, Jerry exhibited a harsh, breathy voice with frequent pitch breaks. He had difficulty sustaining phonation. His intensity sometimes became inaudible towards the end of phrases.

I recommended that Jerry have a laryngeal evaluation. He reported that you were his otolaryngologist and would be making an appointment with you. According to Jerry's request, I have enclosed a copy of his voice evaluation. If you have questions, please contact me.

Sincerely,

John MacGregor, M.S., CCC/SLP
Speech-Language Pathologist

Appendix P

Discrete Trial Baseline Procedure and Recording Sheet

The following illustrates the discrete trial baserating procedure. The example shows how to baserate the correct production of speech sounds. You can adapt it to baserate other target behaviors.

Client: Thomas Tucks   Clinician: Belinda Speaks
Age: 10   Date: 10-10-92
Disorder: Articulation   Session No. 1
Target sound: Initial /s/   Reinforcement: Noncontingent

1.

		Trials	
Target Behaviors		Evoked	Modeled
1.	Sun	–	–
2.	Soup	–	–
3.	Seed	–	–
4.	Soap	–	+
5.	Sink	–	–
6.	Sock	–	+
7.	Suit	–	–

Target Behaviors	Trials	
	Evoked	Modeled
8. Cent	–	–
9. Salt	–	–
10. Sign	–	–
11. Salad	–	–
12. Sofa	–	–
13. Soda	–	–
14. Swing	–	–
15. Syrup	–	–
16. Sunrise	–	–
17. Sweater	–	–
18. Circle	–	–
19. Sand	–	–
20. Sandwich	–	–

Note: (–) = Incorrect; (+) = Correct. Incorrect production of word-initial /s/ on evoked trials: 0%.
Incorrect production on modeled trials: 90%.
(The target phoneme was correctly produced in 2 out of 20 modeled trials).

Index

301